T0249446

Treatment of Colorectal Cancer

Editors

NANCY N. BAXTER
MARCUS J. BURNSTEIN

SURGICAL ONCOLOGY
CLINICS OF NORTH AMERICA

www.surgonc.theclinics.com

Consulting Editor
NICHOLAS J. PETRELLI

January 2014 • Volume 23 • Number 1

ELSEVIER

1600 John F. Kennedy Boulevard • Suite 1800 • Philadelphia, Pennsylvania, 19103-2899

http://www.theclinics.com

SURGICAL ONCOLOGY CLINICS OF NORTH AMERICA Volume 23, Number 1
January 2014 ISSN 1055-3207, ISBN-13: 978-0-323-26414-3

Editor: Jessica McCool
Developmental Editor: Stephanie Carter

Surgical Oncology Clinics of North America (ISSN 1055-3207) is published quarterly by Elsevier Inc., 360 Park Avenue South, New York, NY 10010-1710. Months of publication are January, April, July, and October. Business and Editorial Offices: 1600 John F. Kennedy Blvd., Ste. 1800, Philadelphia, PA 19103-2899. Customer Service Office: 3251 Riverport Lane, Maryland Heights, MO 63043. Periodicals postage paid at New York, NY and additional mailing offices. Subscription prices are $290.00 per year (US individuals), $421.00 (US institutions) $140.00 (US student/resident), $330.00 (Canadian individuals), $533.00 (Canadian institutions), $205.00 (Canadian student/resident), $410.00 (foreign individuals), $533.00 (foreign institutions), and $205.00 (foreign student/resident). Foreign air speed delivery is included in all *Clinics* subscription prices. All prices are subject to change without notice. **POSTMASTER:** Send address changes to *Surgical Oncology Clinics of North America*, Elsevier Health Science Division, Subscription Customer Service, 3251 Riverport Lane, Maryland Heights, MO 63043. **Customer Service: 1-800-654-2452 (US and Canada). 314-447-8871 (outside U.S. and Canada). Fax: 314-447-8029. E-mail: journalscustomerservice-usa@elsevier.com** (for print support); **journalsonline support-usa@elsevier.com** (for online support).

Reprints. For copies of 100 or more, of articles in this publication, please contact the Commercial Reprints Department, Elsevier Inc., 360 Park Avenue South, New York, New York 10010-1710. Tel. 212-633-3874; Fax: 212-633-3820; E-mail: reprints@elsevier.com.

Surgical Oncology Clinics of North America is covered in *MEDLINE/PubMed (Index Medicus)* and *EMBASE/ Excerpta Medica, Current Contents/Clinical Medicine,* and *ISI/BIOMED.*

Printed and bound by CPI Group (UK) Ltd, Croydon, CR0 4YY

Transferred to digital print 2012

Contributors

CONSULTING EDITOR

NICHOLAS J. PETRELLI, MD, FACS
Bank of America Endowed Medical Director, Helen F. Graham Cancer Center at Christiana Care, Newark, Delaware; Professor of Surgery, Thomas Jefferson University, Philadelphia, Pennsylvania

EDITORS

NANCY N. BAXTER, MD, PhD
Associate Professor, Department of Surgery, University of Toronto; Attending Staff, St Michael's Hospital, Toronto, Ontario, Canada

MARCUS J. BURNSTEIN, MD
Associate Professor, Department of Surgery, University of Toronto; Attending Staff, St Michael's Hospital, Toronto, Ontario, Canada

AUTHORS

GERARD BEETS, MD
Department of Surgery, Maastricht University Medical Center, Maastricht, The Netherlands

REGINA BEETS-TAN, MD
Department of Radiology, Maastricht University Medical Center, Maastricht, The Netherlands

CHRISTINE BREZDEN-MASLEY, MD, PhD, FRCPC
Medical Oncologist, Division Head of Hematology/Oncology, St Michael's Hospital; Assistant Professor, Department of Medicine, University of Toronto, Toronto, Ontario, Canada

SIMON J.A. BUCZACKI, MA, MRCS, PhD
Cancer Research UK Clinician Scientist, Cambridge Colorectal Unit, Addenbrooke's Hospital, Cambridge University Hospitals NHS Foundation Trust, Cambridge, United Kingdom

JAMES CHURCH, MBChB, FRACS
Victor Fazio Chair of Colorectal Surgery, Department of Colorectal Surgery, Digestive Diseases Institute, Cleveland Clinic Foundation, Cleveland, Ohio

ROBERT R. CIMA, MD
Professor of Surgery, Division of Colon and Rectal Surgery, Mayo Clinic, Rochester, Minnesota

R. JUSTIN DAVIES, MA, MChir, FRCS (Gen Surg), EBSQ (Coloproctology)
Consultant Colorectal Surgeon, Cambridge Colorectal Unit, Addenbrooke's Hospital, Cambridge University Hospitals NHS Foundation Trust, Cambridge, United Kingdom

FREDERICK DENSTMAN, MD, FASCRS
Helen F. Graham Cancer Center, Christiana Care Health System, Newark, Delaware

DANIEL FISH, MD
Memorial Sloan-Kettering Cancer Center, New York, New York

JULIO GARCIA-AGUILAR, MD, PhD
Chief, Colorectal Service, Department of Surgery, Stuart H.Q. Quan Chair in Colorectal Surgery, Memorial Sloan-Kettering Cancer Center, New York, New York

TORBJÖRN HOLM, MD, PhD
Associate Professor of Surgery, Section of Coloproctology, Department of Surgical Gastroenterology, Karolinska University Hospital, Stockholm, Sweden

KELLIE L. MATHIS, MD
Assistant Professor of Surgery, Division of Colon and Rectal Surgery, Mayo Clinic, Rochester, Minnesota

HEIDI NELSON, MD
Professor of Surgery, Division of Colon and Rectal Surgery, Mayo Clinic, Rochester, Minnesota

P. TERRY PHANG, MD, MSc, FRCSC, FACS
Department of Surgery, St. Paul's Hospital, University of British Columbia, Vancouver, British Columbia, Canada

CHANELE POLENZ, BSc Candidate
University of Waterloo, Ontario, Canada

TUSHAR SAMDANI, MD
Memorial Sloan-Kettering Cancer Center, New York, New York

LARISSA K. TEMPLE, MD, FASC, FRCS(C)
Associate Attending, Colorectal Service, Department of Surgery, Memorial Sloan-Kettering Cancer Center; Associate Professor, Department of Surgery, Weill Cornell Medical College, New York, New York

XIAODONG WANG, MD
Gastrointestinal Surgery Centre, West China Hospital, Sichuan University, Chengdu, Sichuan, China

MARTIN R. WEISER, MD
Department of Surgery, Memorial Sloan–Kettering Cancer Center; Associate Professor, Department of Surgery, Weill Cornell Medical College, New York, New York

Contents

The purpose of most colonoscopies is to detect and treat colorectal neoplasia, preventing or providing early diagnosis of cancer. Basic to this mission is the recognition and diagnosis of neoplasms. Recent data suggest that detection of neoplasia during colonoscopy is suboptimal, resulting in a failure of screening colonoscopy as an efficient strategy for the prevention of cancer. In this article, the ramifications of these observations are examined and their relevance to the practice of colonoscopy considered.

Surgery remains the cornerstone in the multidisciplinary treatment of colon and rectal cancer. Many diagnostic, technical, and adjuvant therapies are known to impact the immediate and long-term oncologic results. Guidelines for appropriate cancer-specific management of colorectal cancer should be adhered to so as to optimize the oncologic outcomes. Similarly, patient-specific surgical outcomes are also linked to many systems-based factors, such as appropriate use of perioperative antibiotics, venous thromboembolism prophylaxis, and avoidance of surgical complications.

The traditional approach to surgical resection of colonic cancer involves removal of the primary tumor together with the associated lymphovascular pedicle. In an attempt to improve oncological outcomes, several groups have recently published data describing improved outcomes with a more radical surgical approach termed complete mesocolic excision (CME) with central vessel ligation (CVL). Here we critically appraise this new surgical advance and discuss other surgical options suggested to offer improvements over current best practice.

There is sufficient level I evidence to support and even recommend laparoscopy as the surgical modality of choice for colon cancer resection.

Controversies in Abdominoperineal Excision

Torbjörn Holm

Abdominoperineal excision (APE) is a necessary operation in many patients with low rectal cancer. Outcomes after this procedure, however, have been variable and often suboptimal. With a new concept of APE, three different types of procedures can be described, based on pelvic and pelvic floor anatomy: intersphincteric APE, extralevator APE (ELAPE), and ischioanal APE. Improved outcomes have been reported after ELAPE but the concept is still controversial and there are disagreements related to the extent of pelvic floor removal, positioning of the patient, and methods of pelvic floor reconstruction.

Management of Complete Response After Chemoradiation in Rectal Cancer

Martin R. Weiser, Regina Beets-Tan, and Gerard Beets

There are an increasing number of reports on nonoperative management of rectal cancer patients who achieve a dramatic response to neoadjuvant therapy. This review discusses the current literature, and describes treatment strategies for patients who have a complete clinical response on follow-up endoscopy after chemoradiotherapy.

Functional Consequences of Colorectal Cancer Management

Daniel Fish and Larissa K. Temple

Functional outcomes of colorectal cancer treatment are an increasingly prominent interest of patients, clinicians, and researchers. The current literature on function after colorectal cancer treatment is difficult to assimilate, with many small, retrospective studies that use a wide variety of nonvalidated measurement tools. Post-treatment dysfunction after rectal cancer therapy is common and often severe. Post-treatment dysfunction is usually less severe for colon cancer patients. Functional outcomes pertinent to colorectal cancer can generally be categorized into three domains: bowel, sexual, and urinary. Several therapies are being explored to improve function, including pharmacologic methods, control and strengthening exercises, and surgical techniques. Further research is needed.

An Approach to the Newly Diagnosed Colorectal Cancer Patient with Synchronous Stage 4 Disease

Frederick Denstman

At initial presentation, 20% to 30% of patients with colon and rectal cancer have detectable metastatic disease. Precise guidelines are lacking for the treatment of this special subset. Most of these patients have only hepatic metastases. Treatment recommendations for these stage 4 patients must take into account characteristics of the primary tumor, the potential resectability of the metastatic disease, and the proper role of chemotherapy and radiation therapy. Because of the tremendous variability of these characteristics, recommendations must be individualized. This article is a basic approach to the treatment of these patients.

Index

SURGICAL ONCOLOGY
CLINICS OF NORTH AMERICA

RELATED INTEREST

Gastroenterology Clinics of North America, September 2013 (Vol. 42, Issue 3)
Colonoscopy and Polypectomy
Charles J. Kahi, MD, *Editor*
Available at: http://www.gastro.theclinics.com/

NOW AVAILABLE FOR YOUR iPhone and iPad

Foreword

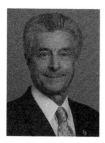

Nicholas J. Petrelli, MD, FACS
Consulting Editor

This issue of the *Surgical Oncology Clinics of North America* is devoted to colorectal cancer. The editors are Nancy N. Baxter, MD, at the University of Toronto, who is a member of the Royal College of Colorectal Surgeons of Canada and staff surgeon in the Department of Surgery at St. Michael's Hospital, and Marcus J. Burnstein, MD, who is an associate professor in the Department of Surgery at the University of Toronto.

This year the American Cancer Society estimates that there will be 102,480 new cases of colorectal cancer and 40,340 new cancer cases of rectal cancer. Colorectal cancer is the third most common cancer in both men and women in the United States. The cancer incidence rates in this disease site have been decreasing for most of the past two decades, which has been attributed to increases in the use of colorectal cancer screening tests inclusive of colonoscopy, which allows for the detection and removal of polyps before they progress to cancer. From 2005 to 2009, incidence rates declined by 4.1% per year among adults 50 years of age and older for whom colorectal screening is recommended and increased by 1.1% per year among those younger than age 50.

In our own state of Delaware, the Colorectal Cancer Screening Program has been a tremendous success. Colorectal cancer screening rates for all Delawareans age 50 years and greater increased from 57% in 2002 to 74% in 2009. In 2008, the disparity between African-Americans and Caucasians for colorectal screening ended with over 90% of the screenings across the state being performed with colonoscopy. The mortality declined by 42% for African-Americans, resulting in a rate almost equal to that among Caucasians in 2009. If the success of the Delaware Colorectal Cancer Screening Program could be performed across the United States, 4,200 fewer African-Americans would get colorectal cancer each year and 2,700 fewer would die as a result. The increased colorectal screening in Delaware, which includes screening through the Delaware Cancer Consortium program and private insurance, saves 8.5 million dollars annually from reduced incidence of cancer and stage shift to cancers requiring less aggressive therapy. This annual savings more than offsets the more than 6 million dollar annual cost of the Cancer Treatment Program that provides universal treatment for all varieties of cancer.

Surg Oncol Clin N Am 23 (2014) ix–x
http://dx.doi.org/10.1016/j.soc.2013.09.007
1055-3207/14/$ – see front matter © 2014 Elsevier Inc. All rights reserved.

surgonc.theclinics.com

I would like to thank Drs Baxter and Burnstein for an outstanding issue of the *Surgical Oncology Clinics of North America*, which updates us about the latest prevention and treatment research in colorectal cancer.

Nicholas J. Petrelli, MD, FACS
Helen F. Graham Cancer Center at Christiana Care
4701 Ogletown-Stanton Road, Suite 1233
Newark, DE 19713, USA

E-mail address:
npetrelli@christianacare.org

Preface

Treatment of Colorectal Cancer

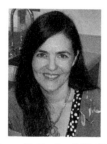 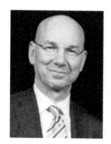

Nancy N. Baxter, MD, PhD Marcus J. Burnstein, MD
Editors

Despite tremendous advances, colorectal cancer remains a hugely important problem and an abundance of important questions about colorectal cancer persist:

- Is the sharp, precision dissection that is so critical and technically challenging in achieving an R0 resection for rectal cancer just as critical for colon cancer?
- Do the higher local and distant recurrence rates following APR for rectal cancer indicate different biology in the distal rectum, or is this a technical problem that is overcome by an extralevator approach to the perineal dissection?
- What local imaging of rectal cancer is optimal for selection of appropriate preoperative and operative management?
- Will MRI fulfill the promise of allowing us to develop a more selective approach to neoadjuvant chemoradiotherapy?
- How should we manage the rectal cancer patient who has a complete response to neoadjuvant chemoradiotherapy?
- Can we do better in the secondary prevention of colorectal cancer?
- Can we do better in the management of stage 4 disease?
- How well are we delivering and ensuring a high quality of care for all patients with colorectal cancer?
- Is there anything left to prove in laparoscopic resection for colon and rectal cancer?
- What is the current state of adjuvant chemotherapy?
- Can we improve the quality of life for patients who survive their treatment for colorectal cancer?

We wanted answers to these questions, and we have collected our most knowledgeable and clear-thinking colleagues to provide them, or at least, to review the

http://dx.doi.org/10.1016/j.soc.2013.09.010
1055-3207/14/$ – see front matter

current, best evidence. They have done an excellent job and we are confident you will agree.

Nancy N. Baxter, MD, PhD
Department of Surgery
University of Toronto
St Michael's Hospital
30 Bond Street, 16CC-040
Toronto, Ontario M5B 1W8, Canada

Marcus J. Burnstein, MD
Department of Surgery
University of Toronto
St Michael's Hospital
30 Bond Street, 16-046
Toronto, Ontario M5B 1W8, Canada

E-mail addresses:
BaxterN@smh.ca (N.N. Baxter)
BURNSTEINM@smh.ca (M.J. Burnstein)

Colonoscopy: What Are We Missing?

James Church, MBChB, FRACS

KEYWORDS

• Colonoscopy • Adenoma • Miss rate • Detection

KEY POINTS

- Missed lesions during colonoscopy are a problem.
- Missed lesions contribute to interval cancers and impair assessment of the stability of the colorectal epithelium.
- Minimizing missed lesions will involve improving colonoscopy quality as defined by completion rates, technique, and accuracy of inspection.
- Improving inspection accuracy means an uncompromising approach to colon cleansing, development of pattern recognition for serrated polyps as well as adenomas, and taking an appropriate amount of time on scope withdrawal.

INTRODUCTION

Colonoscopy has three main roles in the area of colorectal neoplasia. The first is to screen for the disease, preventing it by the detection and removal of potentially premalignant lesions, or providing presymptomatic diagnosis of cancers at an early stage. The second is to diagnose the disease by the investigation of symptoms. The third is to prevent metachronous cancer by the surveillance of patients who already have had a colorectal neoplasm. The efficacy of colonoscopy in fulfilling these roles depends on an accurate examination of the entire colorectal mucosa. This is the rub. In an era of "pay for performance" and a time of increased demand for screening and surveillance colonoscopy, quality has become an important issue. Indices of quality of colonoscopy are now more pragmatic, focused more on what is found than how complete the examination or how satisfied the patient. In this article, the miss rates of colonoscopy are considered and the impact of miss rates on the incidence of colorectal cancer is examined.

BIOLOGY

Before discussing colonoscopy and its ability to detect colorectal neoplasia, it is important to consider the molecular mechanisms by which colorectal neoplasia

The author has nothing to disclose.
Department of Colorectal Surgery, Digestive Diseases Institute, Cleveland Clinic Foundation, Desk A 30, 9500 Euclid Avenue, Cleveland, OH 44195, USA
E-mail address: churchj@ccf.org

Surg Oncol Clin N Am 23 (2014) 1–9
http://dx.doi.org/10.1016/j.soc.2013.09.001
1055-3207/14/$ – see front matter © 2014 Elsevier Inc. All rights reserved.

develops. There are three main ones. Chromosomal instability is the most common, giving rise to 60% of colon cancers and 90% of rectal cancers.[1,2] The accumulation of genetic changes (mutations, hypomethylation, and loss of heterozygosity) is reflected in the mucosa by a progression from small adenomas to larger adenomas to severely dysplastic adenomas to cancer.[3] CpG island methylator phenotype (CIMP) is the second most common, a widespread methylation of CpG promoter islands that causes loss of expression of many genes. When combined with an initial BRAF mutation, such hypermethylation produces advanced serrated polyps (sessile serrated adenomas/polyps [SSA/Ps]) that become severely dysplastic and ultimately malignant.[4] Approximately 18% of colon cancers and 4% of rectal cancers are CIMP-high.[1,2] The third most common mechanism is loss of DNA mismatch repair. This causes mutations throughout the DNA due to single base or loop mismatches at DNA microsatellites, a phenotype known as microsatellite instability (MSI). High levels of MSI can lead to cancer by causing carcinogenic mutations in a variety of genes. Most mutator cancers arise from adenomas, but serrated polyps are also effects of the mechanism. Approximately 18% of colon and 3% of rectal cancers are mutator cancers.[1,2] The most common cause of MSI colon cancers is sporadic hypermethylation of *MLH1*, a DNA mismatch repair gene. Some MSI cancers, however, are due to a germline mutation in 1 of 4 DNA mismatch repair genes, known as Lynch syndrome. Colonoscopy intervenes in the mucosal manifestation of these mechanisms but does nothing to the underlying risk. Patients diagnosed with the hereditary versions of these mechanisms (chromosomal instability = familial adenomatous polyposis, CIMP+ = serrated polyposis, and mutator = Lynch syndrome) need specialized care that takes into account the instability of the colorectal epithelium with a subsequent high risk of colorectal cancer, the risk of extracolonic cancer, and the status of the family. This is best accomplished in the context of a registry.

AIMS OF COLONOSCOPY

The aims of colonoscopy, as far as colorectal cancer is concerned, are to prevent it or, if it is already there, at least to diagnose it early. The aim is not necessarily to remove all polyps regardless of size. The number and types of polyp in the colorectal mucosa are, however, a reflection of the mechanisms active at a molecular level.[5] This is why it is important to be able accurately to document the cumulative numbers of adenomas and serrated polyps. Just as every colorectal cancer has a unique molecular fingerprint, so every colon has a unique blend of molecular changes that either encourage or discourage neoplasia. Recognizing the degree of instability of the colorectal epithelium is a key to designing an appropriate endoscopic surveillance program. Therefore, the aim of colonoscopy is to find every polyp and to remove and biopsy most of the polyps—not because all polyps turn into a cancer (they do not) but because a risk status can then be assigned to the colon that determines the recommended surveillance interval.

COLONOSCOPY AND CANCER PREVENTION

The National Polyp Study caused a big stir in 1993 when it published its initial results showing a considerable reduction in the death rate from colorectal cancer in patients who had their adenomas removed. Compared to three different control groups, the reduction in colorectal cancer incidence rate was 76%, 88%, and 90%.[6] Recently, a longer follow-up of the patients confirmed a reduction in colorectal cancer mortality of 53%.[7] These data are not analyzed by site of the cancers, however. This was reported by Baxter and colleagues[8] in 2009, in a much different kind of study, looking at the integrated results of population-based colonoscopy; a sort of warts and all approach but one that is likely closer to reality than a prospective, randomized poly-pectomy study. They included 10,292 patients who underwent colonoscopy and compared them to 51,460 controls. Colonoscopy was associated with fewer deaths from left-sided colorectal cancer (odds ratio [OR] 0.33) but not with any reduction in deaths from right-sided colon cancer (OR 0.99). These findings have been reproduced by others,[9,10] raising concerns about the performance of colonoscopy and the prob-lem with finding and removing premalignant lesions in the right colon.

MISS RATES

Polyp miss rates are the best way of determining the accuracy of colonoscopy in detecting neoplasia. Most miss rates are determined by tandem colonoscopy, and a selection of recent series is shown in **Table 1**. The absolute miss rates vary but so do study designs. The summary is useful, however, in showing an average adenoma miss rate of rate of 22%, a range from 12% to 26%, and some of the factors influ-encing miss rates. The most influential factor is size. Small polyps are harder to find. Shape makes a difference in that flat or sessile lesions are also a problem. The number of polyps was significant in two studies, showing that if there are two polyps, there is a strong possibility of a third or a fourth. The influence of polyp location was not consistent, with left-sided polyps easier to find in one study but harder in others. Finally, none of the new techniques seemed to make a difference in detection rates—not narrow band imaging, not the third eye retroscope, not high-definition imaging.

ADENOMA DETECTION RATES

Adenoma detection rates (ADRs) are subtly different from miss rates. ADR is usually defined as the proportion of patients with at least one histologically proved adenoma whereas miss rates are defined as the proportion of the total number of adenomas missed. Thus, a patient who has four adenomas represents a tick in the detection rate column if only one is found and removed. The same scenario is an adenoma miss rate of 75%. This demonstrates the fallacy of overall ADR and one of the prob-lems of using it as a quality indicator.[18] More detailed ADRs have been reported to show the average number of adenomas per patient screened and the number of pa-tients with multiple adenomas or serrated polyps. These rates are not generally used, however, as a summary quality indicator. Advanced ADRs are also reported to show the incidence of high-risk lesions that may be expected during screening colonos-copy. Some recent studies are summarized in **Table 2** to give an indication of the

Table 1
Studies of adenoma miss rates

Author, Year	n	Polyps (%)	Adenomas (%)	Significant Factors
Rex et al,[11] 1997	183	—	24	Size, number (>2), side (right > left)
Leufkens et al,[12] 2012	406	25	26	Number (>2), side (left > right)
Heresbach et al,[13] 2008	294	28	20	Side (left > right), shape (sessile/flat > pedunculated), size
Kaltenbach et al,[14] 2008	276	12.6	12.1	Size
Postic et al,[15] 2002	156	—	23	vs surgical specimen
Ahn et al,[16] 2012	149	16.8	17	—
Harrison et al,[17] 2004	100	36.8	33.3	—

Author	n	Overall ADR (%)	ADR Men (%)	ADR Women (%)	Overall Advanced Adenoma (%)	Advanced Adenoma Men (%)	Advanced Adenoma Women (%)
Table 2 Recent studies of adenoma detection rates							
Coe & Wallace,[19] 2013	864	33.7	41.2	25.4	12.2	15.3	8.7
Ferlitsch et al,[20] 2011	44,350	19.7	24.9	14.8	6.3	8.0	4.7
Diamond et al,[21] 2011	17,275	25.3	30.6	20.1			

sort of detection rates that are reported. Both total adenoma detection and detection of advanced adenomas are considerably higher in men than women. Detection rates in patients on surveillance are also higher than those in average risk screening.[22]

Kaminski and colleagues[23] showed that the risk of interval cancer in patients on a colonoscopy screening or surveillance program is related to ADR. This makes sense and confirms ADR as a significant quality measure, a surrogate for the ability of endoscopists to protect patients from cancer.

WHY ARE ADENOMAS MISSED?

Adenomas can be missed because the colon itself is hard to examine (with tortuous twists and turns, frequent bends, marked spasm, and prominent haustral folds), because the examination is incomplete, because preparation is poor, or because the polyps themselves are hard to see. Polyp size is an obvious and important factor in detection, shown by most studies (see **Table 1**).[11] Adenoma shape is also a factor but one that is harder to document. Although flat adenomas can be found in approximately 10% of colonoscopy patients, the miss rate of flat adenomas is hard to assess.[24] The literature reflects this difficulty as variation in incidence of flat adenomas, but Church and colleagues[25] showed that this is as much due to endoscopic definitions as it is to biology. This study established that missed adenomas may actually have been seen, but may not be recognized as neoplasms, and may not be thought to require biopsy or removal. Such a misinterpretation is equivalent to not seeing the lesion at all.

Incomplete examinations are likely to be a problem in population-based series, where the technical ability of colonoscopists is likely to occupy a much larger range than that in reports from specialist units. The significance of incomplete examinations has been established recently by studies of the yield of secondary examinations performed to complete the procedure.[26] Studies of the effectiveness of screening colonoscopy indict incomplete examinations as a reason for failure to protect against right-sided cancers.[8]

SERRATED POLYP DETECTION

Although the gastroenterology community is gradually waking up to the importance of detecting and removing the more advanced types of serrated polyps (SSA/Ps and traditional serrated polyps), study of the ability to detect these important lesions is lagging. SSA/Ps pose special challenges for colonoscopists. They have a low profile, are the same color as the surrounding mucosa, and, even when covered by telltale mucus, require a different form of pattern recognition than the more obvious adenomas. SSA/Ps have only recently been reliably differentiated from other forms of serrated polyp. Studies of serrated polyp detection that accrued data prior to 2006 include hyperplastic and SSA/Ps in the term, *serrated polyps*. Others use *proximal serrated polyps* as a surrogate for SSA/P. **Table 3** shows studies of serrated polyp detection rates. Liang and colleagues[27] showed no correlation with adenoma detection, meaning that just because endoscopists can detect adenomas does not mean that they are good at detecting serrated lesions. Kahi and colleagues,[28] however, did show a good correlation between adenoma and serrated lesion detection, perhaps because the wider range of detection rates allowed for a more sensitive analysis.

The importance of serrated polyps, in particular SSA/Ps, is shown by analyses of interval cancers, presumed missed at index colonoscopy.[32,33] MSI, CIMP, and right-sided location are all over-represented and are all features of cancers arising from SSA/Ps. This is solid evidence that missed SSA/Ps account for a significant proportion of missed cancers.

HIGH-RISK COLONS

The ability of large bowel mucosa to produce neoplastic lesions is dependent on the molecular biology of the epithelial cells and the capacity of epithelial defenses, which varies between patients, according to gender, age, lifestyle, diet, and heredity.[5,34] It is manifest in the number, size, and histology of lesions produced by their colons. High-risk colons can be defined by the cumulative number of adenomas or serrated polyps, by the occurrence of severely dysplastic lesions, by a strong family history suggesting dominant inheritance of a colorectal cancer predisposition, or by the demonstration of a carcinogenic germline mutation. Extremely high risk, such as that conferred by a germline *APC* mutation, leads to prophylactic colectomy. Less severe versions of high risk, or polyp burdens that can be controlled endoscopically, can be managed by aggressive surveillance. The stakes are high, however, and missed lesions have important consequences: early interval cancers.

1. Lynch syndrome: Lynch syndrome is a dominantly inherited cancer predisposition due to a germline mutation in a DNA mismatch repair gene. The adenoma-cancer sequence is accelerated, and adenomas are typically right sided and of low

Table 3
Studies reporting serrated polyp detection rates

Author	n	SDR and Range (%)	PSDR and Range (%)	LSDR (%)	SSA (%)	HP (%)	ADR and Range (%)	Advanced Adenoma (%)
Milan et al,[22] 2008; Liang et al,[27] 2012	3060	13.9 6.4–18.7	—	—	—	—	20.7 13.4–25.8	—
Kahi et al,[28] 2011	6681	—	13 1–18	—	—	—	38 17–47	—
Hetzel et al,[29] 2010	7192	12.5	20.1	—	0.6 0–2.2	11.7 7.7–31.0	22.2 13.5–36.4	—
Leung et al,[30] 2012	1282	—	7.2	2.3	—	—	26.1	10.5
Wu et al,[31] 2013	643	29	—	—	11.0	—	29	8.6

Abbreviations: HP, hyperplastic polyp; LSDR, large serrated polyp detection rate; PSDR, proximal serrated polyp detection rate; SDR, serrated polyp detection rate.

profile. Even yearly colonoscopy may not protect against interval cancers, so consideration must be given to prophylactic colectomy. Stoffel and colleagues[35] assessed adenoma miss rate at 55% in Lynch syndrome.

2. MYH-associated polyposis/attenuated familial adenomatous polyposis: When there are fewer than 100 adenomas, colonoscopic control can be attempted. There are no data on the long-term effectiveness of this but compliant selected patients can be kept cancer free for at least 5 years.[36] Key to success of endoscopic control is not missing advanced lesions.

3. Serrated polyposis: Interval cancers have been reported in this arbitrarily defined syndrome. Polyp numbers rarely indicate prophylactic colectomy, but where the entire syndrome concerns serrated polyps, missed lesions assume a high profile. Surveillance must be aggressive and 6 monthly examinations are reasonable to gain control of the epithelium.[36]

4. Multiple lesions: Here is where miss rates are important and detection rates irrelevant. Defining stability of the colorectal epithelium by cumulative polyp counts is reasonable but depends on accurate detection of all polyps; it is not sufficient to find one adenoma when there are really five. Surveillance depends on risk and risk is reflected in cumulative polyp numbers.

AVOIDING THE MISSED LESION

The variation in polyp detection rates shown in multiple studies reflects several influential factors that can be targeted by endoscopists who wish to minimize missed lesions.

Technique

Colonoscopy is a difficult procedure to perform. The colon is a 6-foot-long muscular tube coiled within a small abdominal cavity. The tube has variable degrees of fixation and its configuration involves unpredictable turns and twists of variable acuity. Insertion techniques seek to shorten the bowel over the colonoscope, so that withdrawal and polypectomy can be controlled, safe, and effective. Effective inspection needs a cooperative and ideally maneuverable patient, with an unhurried, systematic withdrawal. Detection rates are strongly associated with time of withdrawal. Optimal lesion detection demands excellent technique.[37,38]

Pattern Recognition

It is not enough to see a lesion; it must be recognized as a lesion and accurately biopsied or removed. This is easier for adenomas than it is for serrated polyps, but studies of endoscopic definition of polyp histology show that histology is needed for any lesion. Even small lesions are important for what they contribute to definition of the risk of the colorectal epithelium.

Bowel Preparation

Good bowel preparation is essential for an accurate colonoscopy. Inadequate preparation impairs lesion detection.[39] Although the variety of preparations currently available inhibits development of a standard procedure, differences in colorectal physiology between patients demand a targeted approach to bowel lavage. For high-risk colons, the approach to colorectal cleansing must be uncompromising. For average-risk colons, suboptimal preparation should result in shortening of surveillance intervals.

Instrumental and Technical Measures

Various aids to mucosal inspection exist, including chromoendoscopy, narrow band imaging, the third eye retro scope, and magnifying endoscopy.[40–45] The significance of studies examining the effectiveness of these aids is impaired by the arrival of new generations of endoscopes with high-definition optics and enhanced field of view. The control arm keeps changing, so past studies become irrelevant. It is likely, however, that these aids provide a small increment in lesion detection at best. This is often achieved at the cost of increased time and expense of examination. Most improvements will derive from better technique and more time and effort spent inspecting.

Reinforcements

Two sets of eyes are better than one. Recent studies demonstrate that if a nurse or fellow is watching as well as a colonoscopist, more polyps are found.[46,47]

SUMMARY

Missed lesions during colonoscopy are a problem. They contribute to interval cancers and impair assessment of the stability of the colorectal epithelium. Minimizing missed lesions will involve improving colonoscopy quality as defined by completion rates, technique, and accuracy of inspection. Improving inspection accuracy means an uncompromising approach to colon cleansing, development of pattern recognition for serrated polyps as well as adenomas, and taking an appropriate amount of time on scope withdrawal.

REFERENCES

1. Sanchez JA, Krumroy L, Plummer S, et al. Genetic and epigenetic classifications define clinical phenotypes and determine patient outcomes in colorectal cancer. Br J Surg 2009;96:1196–204.
2. Kalady MF, Sanchez JA, Manilich E, et al. Divergent oncogenic changes influence survival differences between colon and rectal adenocarcinomas. Dis Colon Rectum 2009;52:1039–45.
3. Vogelstein B, Kinzler KW. Cancer genes and the pathways they control. Nat Med 2004;10:789–99.
4. Rex DK, Ahnen DJ, Baron JA, et al. Serrated lesions of the colorectum: review and recommendations from an expert panel. Am J Gastroenterol 2012;107: 1315–29.
5. Costedio M, Church J. Pathways of carcinogenesis are reflected in patterns of polyp pathology in patients screened for colorectal cancer. Dis Colon Rectum 2011;54:1224–8.
6. Winawer SJ, Zauber AG, Ho MN, et al. Prevention of colorectal cancer by colonoscopic polypectomy. The National Polyp Study Workgroup. N Engl J Med 1993; 329:1977–81.
7. Zauber AG, Winawer SJ, O'Brien MJ, et al. Colonoscopic polypectomy and long-term prevention of colorectal-cancer deaths. N Engl J Med 2012;366(8):687–96.
8. Baxter NN, Goldwasser MA, Paszat LF, et al. Association of colonoscopy and death from colorectal cancer. Ann Intern Med 2009;150:1–8.
9. Lakoff J, Paszat LF, Saskin R, et al. Risk of developing proximal versus distal colorectal cancer after a negative colonoscopy: a population-based study. Clin Gastroenterol Hepatol 2008;6:1117–21.

10. Singh H, Nugent Z, Demers AA, et al. The reduction in colorectal cancer mortality after colonoscopy varies by site of the cancer. Gastroenterology 2010;139: 1128–37.

11. Rex DK, Cutler CS, Lemmel GT, et al. Colonoscopic miss rates of adenomas determined by back-to-back colonoscopies. Gastroenterology 1997;112(1):24–8.

12. Leufkens AM, van Oijen MG, Vleggaar FP, et al. Factors influencing the miss rate of polyps in a back-to-back colonoscopy study. Endoscopy 2012;44(5): 470–5.

13. Heresbach D, Barrioz T, Lapalus MG, et al. Miss rate for colorectal neoplastic polyps: a prospective multicenter study of back-to-back video colonoscopies. Endoscopy 2008;40(4):284–90.

14. Kaltenbach T, Friedland S, Soetikno R. A randomised tandem colonoscopy trial of narrow band imaging versus white light examination to compare neoplasia miss rates. Gut 2008;57(10):1406–12.

15. Postic G, Lewin D, Bickerstaff C, et al. Colonoscopic miss rates determined by direct comparison of colonoscopy with colon resection specimens. Am J Gastroenterol 2002;97(12):3182–5.

16. Ahn SB, Han DS, Bae JH, et al. The miss rate for colorectal adenoma determined by quality-adjusted, back-to-back colonoscopies. Gut Liver 2012;6(1):64–70.

17. Harrison M, Singh N, Rex DK. Impact of proximal colon retroflexion on adenoma miss rates. Am J Gastroenterol 2004;99(3):519–22.

18. Church J. Adenoma detection rate and the quality of colonoscopy: the sword has two edges. Dis Colon Rectum 2008;51(5):520–3.

19. Coe SG, Wallace MB. Assessment of adenoma detection rate benchmarks in women versus men. Gastrointest Endosc 2013;77(4):631–5.

20. Ferlitsch M, Reinhart K, Pramhas S, et al. Sex-specific prevalence of adenomas, advanced adenomas, and colorectal cancer in individuals undergoing screening colonoscopy. JAMA 2011;306(12):1352–8.

21. Diamond SJ, Enestvedt BK, Jiang Z, et al. Adenoma detection rate increases with each decade of life after 50 years of age. Gastrointest Endosc 2011;74(1): 135–40.

22. Millan MS, Gross P, Manilich E, et al. Adenoma detection rate: the real indicator of quality in colonoscopy. Dis Colon Rectum 2008;51(8):1217–20.

23. Kaminski MF, Regula J, Kraszewska E, et al. Quality indicators for colonoscopy and the risk of interval cancer. N Engl J Med 2010;362:1795–803.

24. Gorgun E, Church J. Flat adenomas of the large bowel: a single endoscopist study. Dis Colon Rectum 2009;52(5):972–7.

25. Church JM, Muto T, Appau K. Flat lesions of the colorectal mucosa: differences in recognition between Japanese and American endoscopists. Dis Colon Rectum 2004;47(9):1462–6.

26. Ridolfi T, Valente M, Church J. Achieving a complete colonic evaluation in patients with incomplete colonoscopy is worth the effort. Dis Colon Rectum 2013; 56:e65–313. http://dx.doi.org/10.1097/DCR.0b013e31828d97c9.

27. Liang J, Kalady MF, Appau K, et al. Serrated polyp detection rate during screening colonoscopy. Colorectal Dis 2012;14(11):1323–7.

28. Kahi CJ, Hewett DG, Norton DL, et al. Prevalence and variable detection of proximal colon serrated polyps during screening colonoscopy. Clin Gastroenterol Hepatol 2011;9(1):42–6.

29. Hetzel JT, Huang CS, Coukos JA, et al. Variation in the detection of serrated polyps in an average risk colorectal cancer screening cohort. Am J Gastroenterol 2010;105(12):2656.

30. Leung WK, Tang V, Lui PC. Detection rates of proximal or large serrated polyps in Chinese patients undergoing screening colonoscopy. J Dig Dis 2012;13(9): 466–71.

31. Wu H, Kravochuck S, Church J. The yield of office colonoscopy: what should a colonoscopists expect to find? Dis Colon Rectum 2013;56:e65–313. http://dx. doi.org/10.1097/DCR.0b013e31828d97c9.

32. Arain MA, Sawhney M, Sheikh S, et al. CIMP status of interval colon cancers: another piece to the puzzle. Am J Gastroenterol 2010;105:1189–95.

33. Shaukat A, Arain M, Thaygarajan B, et al. Is BRAF mutation associated with interval colorectal cancers? Dig Dis Sci 2010;55(8):2352–6.

34. Church JM. Men tend to be neoplasia-prone while women are neoplasia resistant. Surg Endosc 2000;14(12):1162–6.

35. Stoffel EM, Turgeon DK, Stockwell DH, et al, Great Lakes-New England clinical epidemiology and validation center of the early detection research network. Missed adenomas during colonoscopic surveillance in individuals with Lynch Syndrome (hereditary nonpolyposis colorectal cancer). Cancer Prev Res (Phila) 2008;1(6):470–5.

36. Church J. Controlling polyposis with colonoscopy: is it possible? Is it safe? Fam Cancer 2013;12:S81.

37. Rex DK. Colonoscopic withdrawal technique is associated with adenoma miss rates. Gastrointest Endosc 2000;51:33–6.

38. Lee RH, Tang RS, Muthusamy VR, et al. Quality of colonoscopy withdrawal technique and variability in adenoma detection rates (with videos). Gastrointest Endosc 2011;74:128–34.

39. Chokshi RV, Hovis CE, Hollander T, et al. Prevalence of missed adenomas in patients with inadequate bowel preparation on screening colonoscopy. Gastrointest Endosc 2012;75(6):1197–203.

40. Leufkens AM, DeMarco DC, Rastogi A, et al, Third Eye Retroscope Randomized Clinical Evaluation [TERRACE] Study Group. Effect of a retrograde-viewing device on adenoma detection rate during colonoscopy: the TERRACE study. Gastrointest Endosc 2011;73(3):480–9.

41. Ikematsu H, Saito Y, Tanaka S, et al. The impact of narrow band imaging for colon polyp detection: a multicenter randomized controlled trial by tandem colonoscopy. J Gastroenterol 2012;47(10):1099–107.

42. Qumseya BJ, Wallace MB. Advanced colorectal polyp detection techniques. Curr Gastroenterol Rep 2012;14(5):414–20.

43. Dinesen L, Chua TJ, Kaffes AJ. Meta-analysis of narrow-band imaging versus conventional colonoscopy for adenoma detection. Gastrointest Endosc 2012; 75(3):604–11.

44. Aslanian HR, Shieh FK, Chan FW, et al. Nurse observation during colonoscopy increases polyp detection: a randomized prospective study. Am J Gastroenterol 2013;108(2):166–72.

45. Pohl J, Schneider A, Vogell H, et al. Pancolonic chromoendoscopy with indigo carmine versus standard colonoscopy for detection of neoplastic lesions: a randomised two-centre trial. Gut 2011;60(4):485–90.

46. Hashimoto K, Higaki S, Nishiahi M, et al. Does chromoendoscopy improve the colonoscopic adenoma detection rate? Hepatogastroenterology 2010;57(104): 1399–404.

47. Lee CK, Park DI, Lee SH, et al. Participation by experienced endoscopy nurses increases the detection rate of colon polyps during a screening colonoscopy: a multicenter, prospective, randomized study. Gastrointest Endosc 2011;74(5):1094–102.

Quality Assurance in Colon and Rectal Cancer Surgery

Kellie L. Mathis, MD*, Robert R. Cima, MD

KEYWORDS

- Colon cancer • Rectal cancer • Postoperative complications • Surgical outcomes
- Oncologic outcomes • Quality assurance • Prophylactic antibiotics
- VTE prophylaxis

KEY POINTS

- Technical factors impact short-term and long-term outcomes following colorectal cancer surgery. These include appropriate vascular ligation and lymph node harvest, adequate bowel and radial margins, and technical precision within the correct surgical planes.
- Many systems-based factors also affect patient outcomes following colorectal cancer surgery.
- Systems for the appropriate use of venous thromboembolism prophylaxis and perioperative antibiotics have been designed and should be closely adhered to for optimal outcomes.
- Postoperative complications have implications for immediate as well as long-term oncologic outcomes. Attempts should be made to avoid complications where possible and to quickly diagnose and treat them when they do occur.

INTRODUCTION

Surgical resection remains the primary treatment modality for colon and rectal cancer. Short-term and long-term patient outcomes are influenced by a multitude of factors following colorectal cancer surgery. This review discusses technical and systems-based factors that have been shown to affect outcomes in the management of patients with colon and rectal cancer.

TECHNICAL QUALITY FACTORS IN COLORECTAL CANCER SURGERY
Colon Cancer

Lymphadenectomy and vessel ligation

The length of bowel removed is based on the blood supply that drains the tumor-bearing segment of the colon. It is recommended that the proximal and distal margins

The authors have nothing to disclose.
Division of Colon and Rectal Surgery, Mayo Clinic, 200 First Street Southwest, Rochester, MN 55905, USA
* Corresponding author.
E-mail address: mathis.kellie@mayo.edu

are a minimum of 5 cm each.[1,2] There is no survival advantage to removing additional colon beyond that required after vessel ligation.[3–5] The mesentery to the affected segment should be removed en bloc, incorporating the major feeding vessel(s) and the dependent lymphatic-bearing region. Any malignant-appearing lymph nodes (LNs) outside of the boundaries of this envelope of tissue should also be resected if possible. Standard ligation at the origin of the feeding vessel is recommended by the American Society of Colon and Rectal Surgeons[6] because most studies find no survival benefit with high ligation of the feeding vessel. However, at least one large study has suggested that there is an advantage for overall survival and recurrence rate when high vascular ligation is performed in Dukes B and C tumors of the colon and rectum.[7]

There is abundant evidence suggesting that survival improves with increasing LN harvest.[8] A minimum of 12 LNs should be identified and evaluated from the resected colon cancer specimen to allow for accurate staging. The College of American Pathologists suggests that if fewer than 12 LNs are initially identified, additional procedures (such as fat-clearing techniques) should be performed.[9] Patients with N0 disease status but fewer than 12 LNs examined are considered high-risk stage II disease and should be considered for adjuvant chemotherapy.[10]

En bloc resection for T4 lesions
Contiguous structures to which the tumor has adhered or invaded should be removed en bloc with the colon.[2,6] Inflammatory-appearing adhesions between the tumor and other structures are often malignant, and this cannot be differentiated visually. Poeze and colleagues[11] found that patients with T4 disease who underwent en bloc resection of all involved organs had similar survival outcomes to those with T3 disease.

Synchronous cancers
Approximately 5% of patients with a new diagnosis of colon cancer will have a synchronous lesion within the remaining colon/rectum.[12] There is no difference in outcomes between an extended colectomy and 2 separate segmental resections.[13,14]

Prophylactic oophorectomy
The ovaries should be examined at the time of colon resection and removed if suspicious for metastatic disease. There is no clear benefit to removal of normal-appearing ovaries,[15] and prophylactic oophorectomy is not currently recommended.

Laparoscopy
There is an abundance of level I evidence from 4 large multicenter randomized trials consistently showing that laparoscopic colectomy for cancer is associated with equivalent rates of perioperative morbidity and mortality as open colectomy.[16–19] The same trial groups have reported long-term oncologic outcomes and found no differences in survival and recurrence rates.[20–23] Surgeons with training in laparoscopy should offer a minimally invasive approach to patients with colon cancer and no contraindications to laparoscopy.

Adjuvant chemotherapy
Patients with stage III colon cancer should be considered for adjuvant chemotherapy. Multiple large randomized trials have demonstrated a survival benefit in this patient population.[24] The current standard therapy is oxaliplatin with fluoropyrimidine and leucovorin (FOLFOX).[25,26] Data for stage II colon cancer are mixed, but adjuvant chemotherapy should also be considered for patients with high-risk features in the setting of a clinical trial (T4, perforation, lymphovascular involvement, perineural invasion, poorly differentiated histology, fewer than 12 LNs resected).

Rectal Cancer

Staging

Patients with a new diagnosis of rectal cancer should undergo local tumor staging with an endorectal ultrasound or a dedicated magnetic resonance imaging (MRI) study in an effort to define the depth of tumor penetration through the bowel wall, as well as potential regional LN involvement.[27,28] MRI also offers the ability to estimate the circumferential resection margin (CRM). Patients should also undergo staging studies to rule out metastatic disease to the most common sites of metastasis (liver and lung).[27,28]

Neoadjuvant chemoradiation

Neoadjuvant therapy in the form of external beam radiation and administration of fluoropyrimidine chemotherapy is the standard of care for locally advanced (T3–4, N positive) middle and low rectal tumors. In the United States, the radiation is generally given over a 5-week period with approximately 25 fractions followed by surgery 6 to 12 weeks after the completion of radiation.[29,30] Short-course radiotherapy with only 5 fractions in 5 days followed by surgery within 7 days is also used with similar outcomes. Neoadjuvant radiotherapy is preferred over postoperative radiotherapy. No differences in disease-free or overall survival have been established.[30] Radiotherapy plus total mesorectal excision (TME) is associated with improved local recurrence rates compared with TME alone.[31]

Local excision

Local excision has historically been offered to patients who are considered to be too frail to undergo resection. In fit patients, resection of the tumor-bearing rectum and draining LNs is the standard of care. Local excision of a rectal cancer may be considered for patients with T1 lesions in the absence of high-risk histologic features and detectable LN involvement. The National Cancer Comprehensive Network guidelines maintain that when the following features are present, patients can be offered local excision: T1 lesion, well-differentiated or moderately differentiated histology, absence of lymphovascular invasion, absence of perineural invasion, tumor smaller than 3 cm in diameter, and tumor occupies less than one-third the circumference of the rectal lumen.[27] Local recurrence following transanal excision is 8% to 13% in published studies.[32,33]

Vascular ligation

There is no definite oncologic advantage to high ligation of the inferior mesenteric artery[34] except when apical LNs are clinically positive.[35] In a systematic review, Titu and colleagues[36] found that high tie was associated with an increased LN harvest. High ligation of the inferior mesenteric artery as well as the associated vein does allow for significant "lengthening" of the left colon mesentery, facilitating very low colorectal anastomoses.[37]

Total mesorectal excision

Heald was one of the first surgeons to broadcast the importance of a precisely dissected, nonblunt TME.[38] Multiple studies have demonstrated that TME is superior to intra-mesorectal dissection for oncologic outcomes, morbidity, and postoperative function.[39–41] Hida and colleagues[42] described spread of tumor deposits/LNs within the mesorectum extending at least 4 cm distal to the mucosal border of an upper rectal cancer. This evidence led to the current recommendation that all mid and lower rectal tumors be treated with a complete mesorectal excision and all upper rectal cancers be treated with a minimum of a 5-cm mesorectal margin.[27,28,42] Martling and colleagues[43] showed that a national training program for TME in Sweden resulted in increased sphincter-sparing resections, decreased local recurrence, and improved survival following rectal cancer surgery. The quality of the TME specimen is also under scrutiny. Quirke and colleagues[44] showed that the plane of dissection outside the mesorectum versus within the mesorectal fascia is an independent predictor of local recurrence.

Margins

Historically, 5-cm distal margins were required for all rectal cancers.[45] In the modern era, a 2-cm distal margin is suggested to be adequate for middle and low rectal cancers combined with a TME.[27,28,46] Several investigators have shown that a distal margin of 1 cm for very low rectal cancers following neoadjuvant chemoradiotherapy does not affect local recurrence or disease-free survival.[47–49]

The radial margin or CRM is also important. This has been shown to be an independent predictor of recurrence and survival. A CRM of 1 mm or less is associated with a higher local recurrence rate and decreased overall survival, and a CRM of 2 mm is a predictor of local recurrence.[50]

Lymphadenectomy

The recommended extent of lymphadenectomy in the absence of extensive nodal involvement is as described previously in this article with ligation of the superior hemorrhoidal artery and mesorectal excision. Mekenkamp and colleagues[51] suggest that at least 8 LNs are necessary to accurately assign a nodal stage of N0 for rectal cancer. Clinically positive LNs at the base of the inferior mesenteric artery or in the lateral pelvic compartment should be removed if possible. Routine extended lateral pelvic LN dissection has not been shown to offer a survival benefit and is associated with a higher incidence of urinary and sexual dysfunction than TME alone.[52] Fujita and colleagues[53] are conducting a randomized trial comparing TME alone with TME plus lateral LN dissection. Although the oncologic results are pending, they have reported a higher incidence of clinically significant bleeding and longer operative times in the group undergoing extended lymphadenectomy.

Technique for abdominoperineal resection

Positive CRMs, local recurrence, and bowel perforations are more common for abdominoperineal resection (APR) than for sphincter-saving techniques, and survival is lower. Porter and colleagues[54] described an inadvertent perforation rate of 24% in their series of APRs for rectal cancer. Inadvertent perforation was associated with an increased recurrence rate and decreased survival. Others have published similar findings.[55] This has led to a call for change in APR to a cylindrical, extralevator technique. This dissection may be facilitated by placing the patient in the prone jack-knife position for the perianal phase.[56–59]

Laparoscopy

Randomized trials have shown short-term equivalence between the laparoscopic and open techniques for proctectomy.[60,61] Lymph node harvest is equivalent,[62] and the rate of positive CRM is also similar for the 2 techniques.[63]

Data are limited regarding the oncologic outcomes following laparoscopy for rectal cancer. Multiple trials are ongoing, and currently the laparoscopic technique is advised only by surgeons with advanced laparoscopy expertise in the setting of a clinical trial.

SYSTEM QUALITY FACTORS IN COLORECTAL CANCER SURGERY

As previously discussed, there are a number of diagnostic, therapeutic, and technical factors that influence the oncologic outcomes for patients with colorectal cancer.

These can be considered the cancer-specific quality factors. However, quality cancer surgical care is not completely defined by purely oncologic issues. Numerous surgical system issues influence the surgical outcome of the patient with colorectal cancer. Many of these system quality elements are the same for patients undergoing colorectal surgery for benign conditions. However, patients with colorectal cancer may have a worse prognosis if there are adverse outcomes related to failure to follow best practice. In this section, we review some of the major surgical quality process measures, antibiotic use, and venous thromboprophylaxis. Furthermore, we will review the impact of system factors on complications and oncologic outcomes.

APPROPRIATE PROPHYLACTIC ANTIBIOTIC USE

The rapid development and wide distribution of antibiotics during the latter half of the twentieth century led to dramatic antibiotic use in surgical patients. The indiscriminate use of antibiotics in surgery was first noted in the late 1970s when nearly 50% of hospital antibiotic use was related to surgical prophylaxis.[64] The role of prophylactic antibiotics is to obtain therapeutic tissue levels of antibiotics effective against the most common types of organisms encountered during the operative procedure. For colorectal surgery, that would include antibiotic coverage for skin organisms as well as aerobic and anaerobic intestinal flora.

During the 1980s, numerous studies reported that the optimal timing of administration of prophylactic antibiotics was within 60 minutes of incision.[65,66] These studies also demonstrated that prolonged antibiotic use after surgery had no benefit. Although these basic principles of prophylactic antibiotic use were generally adopted nationwide, the antibiotic choices for colorectal surgery were extremely variable and this led to marked differences in surgical site infections (SSIs) within and between institutions complicating the ability to determine a best practice.[67]

To address this wide variation in surgical antibiotic prophylaxis, an attempt was made to study the impact of a standardized regimen of antibiotic selection, timing of administration, and duration of use. A large population-based study was funded by the Centers for Medicare and Medicaid Services (CMS) and conducted in 56 hospitals in Washington State.[68] Using standardized antibiotic protocols and additional elements, SSIs in the participating hospitals were reduced by 27% from an overall of 2.3% to 1.7% after 1 year. The results of this study launched the first series of national surgical quality process measures that have evolved into the CMS Surgical Care Improvement Program (SCIP). Although instituted as national best practices, there have been follow-up analyses in large population studies that have not observed the same reduction in SSIs.[69] However, looking at specifically colorectal surgery, selecting the appropriate antibiotics, with proper administration, including re-dosing and discontinuing them early, have all been associated with a reduction in SSI.[70–72]

The goal of antibiotic prophylaxis is to have therapeutic antibiotic tissue levels while the wound is open not only at the time of incision but also at closure. This is important for colorectal surgery because of the extended duration of colorectal operations. An additional concern in antibiotic prophylaxis is the increasing size of our patients. Duration of operation and patient size influence how prophylactic antibiotics should be dosed and re-dosed. These essential elements are not considered in the national SCIP quality performance measures. However, the importance of appropriate dosing and re-dosing is reflected in the recent surgical prophylaxis guidelines from the major infectious disease, surgical, and pharmacy societies; the guidelines emphasize weight-based dosing within 60 minutes before skin incision and weight-based re-dosing for cases lasting 3 hours or longer, in addition to appropriate antibiotic selection.[73] Re-dosing is especially important for the most commonly used colorectal surgery prophylactic cephalosporin, cefazolin.

The cause of SSIs in colorectal patients is complex and multifactorial. Certainly, appropriate antibiotic use in the perioperative period will not prevent an SSI. Practices that have successfully demonstrated sustainable reductions in colorectal SSIs have implemented a number of standardized protocols addressing many of the contributing factors to SSIs. However, all of these "SSI reduction bundles" closely follow the national antibiotic prophylaxis guidelines for colorectal surgery.

VENOUS THROMBOEMBOLISM PREVENTION

Venous thromboembolism (VTE) is a frequent complication in patients with cancer. The risk of symptomatic VTE is 4 to 7 times higher than the general population seeking medical care and is increased with recent surgery.[74] In patients with colorectal cancer, a VTE increases adjusted incremental health care cost by nearly fourfold during chemotherapy.[75] In patients undergoing major abdominal surgery who do not receive thromboprophylaxis, the rate of VTE ranges between 15% and 30% with a rate of fatal pulmonary embolism of 1%.[76] In an analysis of the American College of Surgeons National Surgical Quality Improvement Program (ACS-NSQIP) dataset, the incidence of postoperative, symptomatic VTE is 22.0 per 1000 for colon cancer and 16.9 per 1000 for rectal cancer, compared with 13.2 per 1000 and 5.5 per 1000, respectively, for benign conditions.[77] Interestingly, despite some initial reports that laparoscopic colectomy is associated with a lower incidence of VTE, in a meta-analysis of randomized controlled trials comparing laparoscopic with open colectomy in patients with cancer, there was no observed difference in VTE rates.[78]

The recommended VTE prophylaxis for patients undergoing colorectal surgery is a combination of lower extremity intermittent pneumatic compression devices (IPC) with chemical prophylaxis.[79] The recommended chemical prophylaxis is either unfractionated heparin administered 3 times a day or therapeutic low molecular weight heparin (LMWH). These therapies have been shown in patients with abdominal and pelvic malignancies to be equally efficacious with no difference in postoperative bleeding complications.[80] Although a combination therapy including both mechanical and chemical prophylaxis is recommended for colorectal surgery patients, the key component is the chemical prophylaxis. In a randomized controlled trial of LMWH and IPC versus IPC alone in more than 1000 patients undergoing abdominal surgery, the combined use of LMWH and IPC reduced the VTE rate by nearly 70%.[81]

Of course, the primary concern of VTE chemoprophylaxis is a possible increased risk of postoperative bleeding events. In the Enoxaparin and Cancer (ENOXACAN) trial comparing standard unfractionated heparin to LMWH there were similar rates of overall bleeding and major bleeding in both arms, about 17% and 3%, respectively.[80] A systematic review of chemical VTE prophylaxis in patients participating in randomized controlled surgical oncology trials revealed a significant benefit compared with mechanical prophylaxis.[82] The overall rate of bleeding complications that required discontinuation of chemical prophylaxis was 3%. In subsequent studies looking at only colorectal surgery patients, the associated bleeding rates, minor and major events, were in the 3% to 10% range.[83–85] In a large population-based study of colorectal patients in hospitals that used chemoprophylaxis and those that used only mechanical prophylaxis, the chemoprophylaxis hospitals had significantly fewer symptomatic VTE complications and similar or lower bleeding complications.[86] This finding has been demonstrated in additional studies.[84,85] In the large Canadian randomized trial comparing the efficacy of low-dose unfractionated heparin with

LMWH, the rates of bleeding requiring reoperation were 0.2% and 0.3%, respectively.[84] The evidence clearly supports the use of VTE chemoprophylaxis in colorectal surgery patients in the perioperative hospitalization period and this has become a national quality process measure. There is increasing evidence that these patients may significantly benefit from continued VTE chemoprophylaxis after discharge from hospital.

In an analysis of more than 68,000 newly diagnosed patients with colorectal cancer in California, the incidence of VTE within 2 years of diagnosis was 3.1%.[87] Most VTE events occurred within 6 months of diagnosis, more than 30% occurring within 2 months of operation. The presence of a VTE within the first year after diagnosis was a major predictor of death. With the increased use of laparoscopy and postoperative clinical pathways leading to decreased length of stay, the duration of VTE chemoprophylaxis is also decreasing. Increasingly, follow-up data are demonstrating that many VTE complications are being diagnosed after the patient leaves the hospital. According to the ACS-NSQIP data set, more than a third of all colorectal cancer VTE episodes are detected after discharge.[77] Furthermore, the symptomatic patients with VTE diagnosed after discharge from the hospital as compared with those diagnosed in the immediate perioperative period are more likely to have a recurrent VTE in the year after their surgery.[88] The relatively high rate of postdischarge VTE events and the significant morbidity associated with them has prompted investigation of longer VTE prophylaxis. The most recent Cochrane review on the subject of extended thromboprophylaxis after abdominal or pelvic surgery using LMWH concluded that use of prophylaxis for 4 weeks after surgery significantly reduced postdischarge events without an increase in bleeding complications.[89] Prolonged postoperative VTE prophylaxis resulted in a significant reduction in postdischarge symptomatic VTEs from 1.7% to 0.2%, with no difference in associated postoperative bleeding events.

THE IMPACT OF POSTOPERATIVE COMPLICATIONS

Complications have a profound negative impact on the health care system from both a resource utilization and economic point of view. In a study using the initial private-sector NSQIP data set to analyze the cost of complications, a major postoperative complication resulted in an average of $12,000 in additional hospital costs after adjusting for patient characteristics.[90] Infectious complications more than doubled the cost, whereas thromboembolic events increased the cost by more than 6 times the baseline care cost. Although in-patient costs during the initial hospitalization are increased with complications, another substantial problem is the impact of readmissions to address complications. In the ACS-NSQIP dataset, colectomy patients are the most commonly readmitted patients by volume of procedures for the 20 most commonly performed operations.[91] The 30-day readmission rate for colectomy patients was 13.4%. In those patients who had a postoperative complication during the 30-day follow-up after surgery, 53% had a readmission, whereas only 5% with no surgical complication required readmission. The evidence demonstrates that avoiding surgical complications has both patient and economic benefits and there is also evidence to suggest that complications can have a negative impact on oncologic outcomes.

There are conflicting data on the impact of anastomotic leaks and associated infections on the oncologic outcomes for colorectal cancer. McArdle and colleagues[92] analyzed the 5-year survival of more than 2000 patients with colorectal cancer operated on between 1991 and 1994. They found that those with an intra-abdominal leak had significantly lower 5-year survival than those without such a complication when adjusted for stage. In a subsequent study of 1580 patients who underwent curative resection for colorectal cancer, an anastomotic complication was an independent risk factor for decreased 5-year survival and, in the case of rectal cancer, a risk factor for local recurrence.[93] These investigators also examined the impact of overall postoperative complications and found that the presence of a major complication was associated with decreased 5-year survival compared with patients who did not have postoperative complications.[94] Not all studies have demonstrated such an association.[95] In a recent meta-analysis evaluating the impact of anastomotic complications after colorectal cancer surgery, Mirnezami and colleagues[96] evaluated studies that included more than 21,000 patients and found a strong association between an anastomotic complication and worse overall cancer-specific survival. The mechanism responsible for these observations is unknown, but most investigators posit an interaction with a weakened patient's immune system.

SUMMARY

Surgery plays a central role in the care of the patient with colorectal cancer. Quality outcomes are defined by technical, oncologic, and system of care issues. Short-term and long-term patient outcomes have been linked directly to many technical factors, such as adequacy of margins and LN harvest, as well as to adherence to correct surgical planes. Ensuring proper systems of care and adherence to evidence-based best practices in the postoperative period is also important for the uneventful recovery of the postoperative patient with colorectal cancer. Ensuring operative techniques to minimize complications also appears to improve oncologic outcomes.

REFERENCES

1. Park IJ, Choi GS, Kang BM, et al. Lymph node metastasis patterns in right-sided colon cancers: is segmental resection of these tumors oncologically safe? Ann Surg Oncol 2009;16:1501–6.
2. Nelson H, Petrelli N, Carlin A, et al. Guidelines 2000 for colon and rectal cancer surgery. J Natl Cancer Inst 2001;93:583–96.
3. Secco GB, Ravera G, Gasparo A, et al. Segmental resection, lymph nodes dissection and survival in patients with left colon cancer. Hepatogastroenterology 2007;54:422–6.
4. Rouffet F, Hay JM, Vacher B, et al. Curative resection for left colonic carcinoma: hemicolectomy vs. segmental colectomy. A prospective, controlled, multicenter trial. French Association for Surgical Research. Dis Colon Rectum 1994;37:651–9.
5. Di Cataldo A, La Greca G, Lanteri R, et al. Cancer of the sigmoid colon: left hemicolectomy or sigmoidectomy? Int Surg 2007;92:10–4.
6. Chang GJ, Kaiser AM, Mills S, et al. Practice parameters for the management of colon cancer. Dis Colon Rectum 2012;55:831–43.
7. Slanetz CA Jr, Grimson R. Effect of high and intermediate ligation on survival and recurrence rates following curative resection of colorectal cancer. Dis Colon Rectum 1997;40:1205–18 [discussion: 1218–9].
8. Chang GJ, Rodriguez-Bigas MA, Skibber JM, et al. Lymph node evaluation and survival after curative resection of colon cancer: systematic review. J Natl Cancer Inst 2007;99:433–41.
9. Compton CC. Key issues in reporting common cancer specimens: problems in pathologic staging of colon cancer. Arch Pathol Lab Med 2006;130:318–24.

10. Engstrom PF, Arnoletti JP, Benson AB 3rd, et al. NCCN clinical practice guidelines in oncology: colon cancer. J Natl Compr Canc Netw 2009;7:778–831.
11. Poeze M, Houbiers JG, van de Velde CJ, et al. Radical resection of locally advanced colorectal cancer. Br J Surg 1995;82:1386–90.
12. Kim MS, Park YJ. Detection and treatment of synchronous lesions in colorectal cancer: the clinical implication of perioperative colonoscopy. World J Gastroenterol 2007;13:4108–11.
13. Whelan RL, Wong WD, Goldberg SM, et al. Synchronous bowel anastomoses. Dis Colon Rectum 1989;32:365–8.
14. Holubar SD, Wolff BG, Poola VP, et al. Multiple synchronous colonic anastomoses: are they safe? Colorectal Dis 2010;12:135–40.
15. Sielezneff I, Salle E, Antoine K, et al. Simultaneous bilateral oophorectomy does not improve prognosis of postmenopausal women undergoing colorectal resection for cancer. Dis Colon Rectum 1997;40:1299–302.
16. A comparison of laparoscopically assisted and open colectomy for colon cancer. N Engl J Med 2004;350:2050–9.
17. Guillou PJ, Quirke P, Thorpe H, et al. Short-term endpoints of conventional versus laparoscopic-assisted surgery in patients with colorectal cancer (MRC CLASICC trial): multicentre, randomised controlled trial. Lancet 2005;365:1718–26.
18. Hewett PJ, Allardyce RA, Bagshaw PF, et al. Short-term outcomes of the Australasian randomized clinical study comparing laparoscopic and conventional open surgical treatments for colon cancer: the ALCCaS trial. Ann Surg 2008;248:728–38.
19. Veldkamp R, Kuhry E, Hop WC, et al. Laparoscopic surgery versus open surgery for colon cancer: short-term outcomes of a randomised trial. Lancet Oncol 2005;6:477–84.
20. Bagshaw PF, Allardyce RA, Frampton CM, et al. Long-term outcomes of the Australasian randomized clinical trial comparing laparoscopic and conventional open surgical treatments for colon cancer: the Australasian Laparoscopic Colon Cancer Study trial. Ann Surg 2012;256:915–9.
21. Fleshman J, Sargent DJ, Green E, et al. Laparoscopic colectomy for cancer is not inferior to open surgery based on 5-year data from the COST Study Group trial. Ann Surg 2007;246:655–62 [discussion: 662–4].
22. Jayne DG, Thorpe HC, Copeland J, et al. Five-year follow-up of the Medical Research Council CLASICC trial of laparoscopically assisted versus open surgery for colorectal cancer. Br J Surg 2010;97:1638–45.
23. Buunen M, Veldkamp R, Hop WC, et al. Survival after laparoscopic surgery versus open surgery for colon cancer: long-term outcome of a randomised clinical trial. Lancet Oncol 2009;10:44–52.
24. Sargent D, Sobrero A, Grothey A, et al. Evidence for cure by adjuvant therapy in colon cancer: observations based on individual patient data from 20,898 patients on 18 randomized trials. J Clin Oncol 2009;27:872–7.
25. Andre T, Boni C, Navarro M, et al. Improved overall survival with oxaliplatin, fluorouracil, and leucovorin as adjuvant treatment in stage II or III colon cancer in the MOSAIC trial. J Clin Oncol 2009;27:3109–16.
26. Kuebler JP, Wieand HS, O'Connell MJ, et al. Oxaliplatin combined with weekly bolus fluorouracil and leucovorin as surgical adjuvant chemotherapy for stage II and III colon cancer: results from NSABP C-07. J Clin Oncol 2007;25:2198–204.
27. Benson AB 3rd, Bekaii-Saab T, Chan E, et al. Rectal cancer. J Natl Compr Canc Netw 2012;10:1528–64.

28. Monson JR, Weiser MR, Buie WD, et al. Practice parameters for the management of rectal cancer (revised). Dis Colon Rectum 2013;56:535–50.

29. Bosset JF, Collette L, Calais G, et al. Chemotherapy with preoperative radiotherapy in rectal cancer. N Engl J Med 2006;355:1114–23.

30. Sauer R, Becker H, Hohenberger W, et al. Preoperative versus postoperative chemoradiotherapy for rectal cancer. N Engl J Med 2004;351:1731–40.

31. Kapiteijn E, Marijnen CA, Nagtegaal ID, et al. Preoperative radiotherapy combined with total mesorectal excision for resectable rectal cancer. N Engl J Med 2001;345:638–46.

32. Greenberg JA, Shibata D, Herndon JE 2nd, et al. Local excision of distal rectal cancer: an update of cancer and leukemia group B 8984. Dis Colon Rectum 2008;51:1185–91 [discussion: 1191–4].

33. Nash GM, Weiser MR, Guillem JG, et al. Long-term survival after transanal excision of T1 rectal cancer. Dis Colon Rectum 2009;52:577–82.

34. Cirocchi R, Trastulli S, Farinella E, et al. High tie versus low tie of the inferior mesenteric artery in colorectal cancer: a RCT is needed. Surg Oncol 2012;21: e111–23.

35. Kanemitsu Y, Hirai T, Komori K, et al. Survival benefit of high ligation of the inferior mesenteric artery in sigmoid colon or rectal cancer surgery. Br J Surg 2006; 93:609–15.

36. Titu LV, Tweedle E, Rooney PS, et al. High tie of the inferior mesenteric artery in curative surgery for left colonic and rectal cancers: a systematic review. Dig Surg 2008;25(2):148–57.

37. Thum-Umnuaysuk S, Boonyapibal A, Geng YY, et al. Lengthening of the colon for low rectal anastomosis in a cadaveric study: how much can we gain? Tech Coloproctol 2013;17(4):377–81.

38. Heald RJ, Husband EM, Ryall RD. The mesorectum in rectal cancer surgery—the clue to pelvic recurrence? Br J Surg 1982;69:613–6.

39. Bosch SL, Nagtegaal ID. The importance of the pathologist's role in assessment of the quality of the mesorectum. Curr Colorectal Cancer Rep 2012;8:90–8.

40. Cecil TD, Sexton R, Moran BJ, et al. Total mesorectal excision results in low local recurrence rates in lymph node-positive rectal cancer. Dis Colon Rectum 2004; 47:1145–9 [discussion: 1149–50].

41. Heald RJ, Ryall RD. Recurrence and survival after total mesorectal excision for rectal cancer. Lancet 1986;1:1479–82.

42. Hida J, Yasutomi M, Maruyama T, et al. Lymph node metastases detected in the mesorectum distal to carcinoma of the rectum by the clearing method: justification of total mesorectal excision. J Am Coll Surg 1997;184:584–8.

43. Martling AL, Holm T, Rutqvist LE, et al. Effect of a surgical training programme on outcome of rectal cancer in the County of Stockholm. Stockholm Colorectal Cancer Study Group, Basingstoke Bowel Cancer Research Project. Lancet 2000;356:93–6.

44. Quirke P, Steele R, Monson J, et al. Effect of the plane of surgery achieved on local recurrence in patients with operable rectal cancer: a prospective study using data from the MRC CR07 and NCIC-CTG CO16 randomised clinical trial. Lancet 2009;373:821–8.

45. Williams NS, Dixon MF, Johnston D. Reappraisal of the 5 centimetre rule of distal excision for carcinoma of the rectum: a study of distal intramural spread and of patients' survival. Br J Surg 1983;70:150–4.

46. Wolmark N, Fisher B. An analysis of survival and treatment failure following abdominoperineal and sphincter-saving resection in Dukes' B and C rectal

carcinoma. A report of the NSABP clinical trials. National Surgical Adjuvant Breast and Bowel Project. Ann Surg 1986;204:480–9.

47. Guillem JG, Chessin DB, Shia J, et al. A prospective pathologic analysis using whole-mount sections of rectal cancer following preoperative combined modality therapy: implications for sphincter preservation. Ann Surg 2007;245:88–93.

48. Kuvshinoff B, Maghfoor I, Miedema B, et al. Distal margin requirements after preoperative chemoradiotherapy for distal rectal carcinomas: are < or = 1 cm distal margins sufficient? Ann Surg Oncol 2001;8:163–9.

49. Mezhir JJ, Shia J, Riedel E, et al. Whole-mount pathologic analysis of rectal cancer following neoadjuvant therapy: implications of margin status on long-term oncologic outcome. Ann Surg 2012;256:274–9.

50. Nagtegaal ID, Marijnen CA, Kranenbarg EK, et al. Circumferential margin involvement is still an important predictor of local recurrence in rectal carcinoma: not one millimeter but two millimeters is the limit. Am J Surg Pathol 2002;26:350–7.

51. Mekenkamp LJ, van Krieken JH, Marijnen CA, et al. Lymph node retrieval in rectal cancer is dependent on many factors—the role of the tumor, the patient, the surgeon, the radiotherapist, and the pathologist. Am J Surg Pathol 2009;33:1547–53.

52. Georgiou P, Tan E, Gouvas N, et al. Extended lymphadenectomy versus conventional surgery for rectal cancer: a meta-analysis. Lancet Oncol 2009;10:1053–62.

53. Fujita S, Akasu T, Mizusawa J, et al. Postoperative morbidity and mortality after mesorectal excision with and without lateral lymph node dissection for clinical stage II or stage III lower rectal cancer (JCOG0212): results from a multicentre, randomised controlled, non-inferiority trial. Lancet Oncol 2012;13:616–21.

54. Porter GA, O'Keefe GE, Yakimets WW. Inadvertent perforation of the rectum during abdominoperineal resection. Am J Surg 1996;172:324–7.

55. Slanetz CA Jr. The effect of inadvertent intraoperative perforation on survival and recurrence in colorectal cancer. Dis Colon Rectum 1984;27:792–7.

56. Holm T, Ljung A, Haggmark T, et al. Extended abdominoperineal resection with gluteus maximus flap reconstruction of the pelvic floor for rectal cancer. Br J Surg 2007;94:232–8.

57. Marr R, Birbeck K, Garvican J, et al. The modern abdominoperineal excision: the next challenge after total mesorectal excision. Ann Surg 2005;242:74–82.

58. Nagtegaal ID, van de Velde CJ, Marijnen CA, et al. Low rectal cancer: a call for a change of approach in abdominoperineal resection. J Clin Oncol 2005;23:9257–64.

59. West NP, Finan PJ, Anderin C, et al. Evidence of the oncologic superiority of cylindrical abdominoperineal excision for low rectal cancer. J Clin Oncol 2008;26:3517–22.

60. Jayne DG, Guillou PJ, Thorpe H, et al. Randomized trial of laparoscopic-assisted resection of colorectal carcinoma: 3-year results of the UK MRC CLASICC Trial Group. J Clin Oncol 2007;25:3061–8.

61. van der Pas MH, Haglind E, Cuesta MA, et al. Laparoscopic versus open surgery for rectal cancer (COLOR II): short-term outcomes of a randomised, phase 3 trial. Lancet Oncol 2013;14:210–8.

62. Ng KH, Ng DC, Cheung HY, et al. Laparoscopic resection for rectal cancers: lessons learned from 579 cases. Ann Surg 2009;249:82–6.

63. Aziz O, Constantinides V, Tekkis PP, et al. Laparoscopic versus open surgery for rectal cancer: a meta-analysis. Ann Surg Oncol 2006;13:413–24.

64. Shapiro M, Townsend TR, Rosner B, et al. Use of antimicrobial drugs in general hospitals: patterns of prophylaxis. N Engl J Med 1979;301:351–5.

65. Classen DC, Evans RS, Pestotnik SL, et al. The timing of prophylactic administration of antibiotics and the risk of surgical-wound infection. N Engl J Med 1992; 326:281–6.

66. Crossley K, Gardner LC. Antimicrobial prophylaxis in surgical patients. JAMA 1981;245:722–6.

67. Silver A, Eichorn A, Kral J, et al. Timeliness and use of antibiotic prophylaxis in selected inpatient surgical procedures. The Antibiotic Prophylaxis Study Group. Am J Surg 1996;171:548–52.

68. Dellinger EP, Hausmann SM, Bratzler DW, et al. Hospitals collaborate to decrease surgical site infections. Am J Surg 2005;190:9–15.

69. Stulberg JJ, Delaney CP, Neuhauser DV, et al. Adherence to surgical care improvement project measures and the association with postoperative infections. JAMA 2010;303:2479–85.

70. Ho VP, Barie PS, Stein SL, et al. Antibiotic regimen and the timing of prophylaxis are important for reducing surgical site infection after elective abdominal colorectal surgery. Surg Infect (Larchmt) 2011;12:255–60.

71. Nguyen N, Yegiyants S, Kaloostian C, et al. The Surgical Care Improvement project (SCIP) initiative to reduce infection in elective colorectal surgery: which performance measures affect outcome? Am Surg 2008;74:1012–6.

72. Suehiro T, Hirashita T, Araki S, et al. Prolonged antibiotic prophylaxis longer than 24 hours does not decrease surgical site infection after elective gastric and colorectal surgery. Hepatogastroenterology 2008;55:1636–9.

73. Bratzler DW, Dellinger EP, Olsen KM, et al. Clinical practice guidelines for antimicrobial prophylaxis in surgery. Am J Health Syst Pharm 2013;70:195–283.

74. Lyman GH, Khorana AA, Falanga A. Thrombosis and cancer. Am Soc Clin Oncol Educ Book 2013;2013:337–45.

75. Khorana AA, Dalal MR, Lin J, et al. Health care costs associated with venous thromboembolism in selected high-risk ambulatory patients with solid tumors undergoing chemotherapy in the United States. Clinicoecon Outcomes Res 2013;5:101–8.

76. Geerts WH, Pineo GF, Heit JA, et al. Prevention of venous thromboembolism: the Seventh ACCP Conference on Antithrombotic and Thrombolytic Therapy. Chest 2004;126:338S–400S.

77. Reinke CE, Karakousis GC, Hadler RA, et al. Incidence of venous thromboembolism in patients undergoing surgical treatment for malignancy by type of neoplasm: an analysis of ACS-NSQIP data from 2005 to 2010. Surgery 2012;152:186–92.

78. Cui G, Wang X, Yao W, et al. Incidence of postoperative venous thromboembolism after laparoscopic versus open colorectal cancer surgery: a meta-analysis. Surg Laparosc Endosc Percutan Tech 2013;23:128–34.

79. Gould MK, Garcia DA, Wren SM, et al. Prevention of VTE in nonorthopedic surgical patients: Antithrombotic Therapy and Prevention of Thrombosis, 9th ed: American College of Chest Physicians Evidence-Based Clinical Practice Guidelines. Chest 2012;141:e227S–77S.

80. Efficacy and safety of enoxaparin versus unfractionated heparin for prevention of deep vein thrombosis in elective cancer surgery: a double-blind randomized multicentre trial with venographic assessment. ENOXACAN Study Group. Br J Surg 1997;84:1099–103.

81. Turpie AG, Bauer KA, Caprini JA, et al. Fondaparinux combined with intermittent pneumatic compression vs. intermittent pneumatic compression alone for

prevention of venous thromboembolism after abdominal surgery: a randomized, double-blind comparison. J Thromb Haemost 2007;5:1854–61.

82. Leonardi MJ, McGory ML, Ko CY. A systematic review of deep venous thrombosis prophylaxis in cancer patients: implications for improving quality. Ann Surg Oncol 2007;14:929–36.

83. Henke PK, Arya S, Pannucci C, et al. Procedure-specific venous thromboembolism prophylaxis: a paradigm from colectomy surgery. Surgery 2012;152:528–34 [discussion: 534–6].

84. McLeod RS, Geerts WH, Sniderman KW, et al. Subcutaneous heparin versus low-molecular-weight heparin as thromboprophylaxis in patients undergoing colorectal surgery: results of the Canadian colorectal DVT prophylaxis trial: a randomized, double-blind trial. Ann Surg 2001;233:438–44.

85. Sanderson B, Hitos K, Fletcher JP. Venous thromboembolism following colorectal surgery for suspected or confirmed malignancy. Thrombosis 2011;2011: 828030.

86. Kwon S, Meissner M, Symons R, et al. Perioperative pharmacologic prophylaxis for venous thromboembolism in colorectal surgery. J Am Coll Surg 2011;213: 596–603, 603.e1.

87. Alcalay A, Wun T, Khatri V, et al. Venous thromboembolism in patients with colorectal cancer: incidence and effect on survival. J Clin Oncol 2006;24:1112–8.

88. Toledano TH, Kondal D, Kahn SR, et al. The occurrence of venous thromboembolism in cancer patients following major surgery. Thromb Res 2013;131:e1–5.

89. Rasmussen MS, Jorgensen LN, Wille-Jorgensen P. Prolonged thromboprophylaxis with low molecular weight heparin for abdominal or pelvic surgery. Cochrane Database Syst Rev 2009;(1):CD004318.

90. Dimick JB, Chen SL, Taheri PA, et al. Hospital costs associated with surgical complications: a report from the private-sector National Surgical Quality Improvement Program. J Am Coll Surg 2004;199:531–7.

91. Lawson EH, Hall BL, Louie R, et al. Association between occurrence of a postoperative complication and readmission: implications for quality improvement and cost savings. Ann Surg 2013;258:10–8.

92. McArdle CS, McMillan DC, Hole DJ. Impact of anastomotic leakage on long-term survival of patients undergoing curative resection for colorectal cancer. Br J Surg 2005;92:1150–4.

93. Law WL, Choi HK, Lee YM, et al. Anastomotic leakage is associated with poor long-term outcome in patients after curative colorectal resection for malignancy. J Gastrointest Surg 2007;11:8–15.

94. Law WL, Choi HK, Lee YM, et al. The impact of postoperative complications on long-term outcomes following curative resection for colorectal cancer. Ann Surg Oncol 2007;14:2559–66.

95. Smith JD, Butte JM, Weiser MR, et al. Anastomotic leak following low anterior resection in stage IV rectal cancer is associated with poor survival. Ann Surg Oncol 2013;20(8):2641–6.

96. Mirnezami A, Mirnezami R, Chandrakumaran K, et al. Increased local recurrence and reduced survival from colorectal cancer following anastomotic leak: systematic review and meta-analysis. Ann Surg 2011;253:890–9.

Colon Resection
Is Standard Technique Adequate?

Simon J.A. Buczacki, MA, MRCS, PhD,
R. Justin Davies, MA, MChir, FRCS (Gen Surg), EBSQ(Coloproctology)*

KEYWORDS

- Colon cancer • Surgery • Lymph node • Complete mesocolic excision

KEY POINTS

- The principles behind colon cancer resections have changed little over the past few decades.
- Recent data suggest improved outcomes in colon cancer surgery with wider resections of lymphovascular pedicles along defined anatomic planes compared with traditional approaches.
- There are no definitive data demonstrating biologically why larger lymph node yields or identification equates to improved oncological outcomes.
- Intratumoral and intertumoral clonal heterogeneity likely confounds many surgical studies.

INTRODUCTION

Colorectal cancer is the third most common cancer worldwide, accounting for approximately 600,000 deaths per annum (CRUK Cancer Stats: http://www.cancerresearchuk.org/cancer-info/cancerstats/types/bowel/mortality/). The potentially curative primary treatment for patients with both colon and rectal cancer remains surgery. Adjuvant treatment with chemotherapy provides additional benefit for those patients with more advanced colonic tumors.

Over the past few decades, there have been significant improvements in the treatment of patients with colonic and rectal cancers. In rectal cancer, the role of earlier diagnosis, improved preoperative staging, neoadjuvant therapy, total mesorectal excision, and laparoscopic surgery have improved outcomes from oncological and patient recovery perspectives. Of these, arguably the most important for the surgeon was the advent of total mesorectal excision (TME) by Heald and Ryall.[1]

The authors have no competing interests.
Cambridge Colorectal Unit, Addenbrooke's Hospital, Cambridge University Hospitals NHS Foundation Trust, Cambridge Biomedical Campus, Hills Road, Cambridge, CB2 0QQ, UK
* Corresponding author.
E-mail address: justin.davies@addenbrookes.nhs.uk

Current thinking is that colonic tumors spread via hematogenous, lymphatic, and possibly perineural routes, with the lymphatics anatomically following the arterial supply. Current practice is to excise a proportion of the draining lymphatic bed to accurately stage the cancer and also clear possible lymphatic metastases.[2] Recently, significant debate has centered on the degree of lymphatic clearance required; several reports have demonstrated improved oncologic outcomes with wider lymphovascular resections compared with current standard practice. Whether these improved outcomes are secondary to improved lymph node yield or an alternative technical effect has not yet been ascertained.

CURRENT SURGICAL PRACTICE FOR COLONIC RESECTION

The traditional approach to surgical colon cancer resection involves removal of the primary tumor with adequate proximal and distal resection margins, and a clear circumferential resection margin (which may require en bloc resection of the abdominal wall or other viscera) together with an anatomically defined mesenteric lymphovascular pedicle. These operations may be performed via either a traditional open approach or laparoscopically. It has now been shown by a wide number of studies, including large randomized controlled trials (RCT), such as COST,[3] CLASICC,[4] and COLOR,[5] that oncological outcomes from laparoscopic colonic surgery are equivalent to open surgery. The necessity to include resection of the lymphovascular mesentery is based on the tenet that in addition to hematogeneous spread, colonic tumors most commonly spread initially via the lymphatic system, which anatomically follows the colonic arterial supply. Historically it is held that en bloc lymph node resection is necessary not only for staging (Cady-Fisher) but also to reduce tumor burden (Halsted). The Cady-Fisher model of cancer progression proposes that systemic spread occurs as an early event in cancer development, whereas the Halsted theory suggests a more stepwise progression in the development of metastases. More contemporary views on the role of lymphadenectomy have seen it purely for staging purposes, the results of which effect management by defining adjuvant treatment options. Generally speaking, adjuvant chemotherapy is reserved for those patients with lymph node involvement (stage III/IV) or poor prognosis stage II cancers. Inadequate assessment of lymph nodes for malignancy will theoretically lead to understaging, resulting in increased mortality through undertreatment. Understaging may be consequent on either the surgeon not removing enough lymph nodes or the pathologist not identifying and examining all lymph nodes present in the specimen. In relation to the latter, various options have been evaluated to increase the identification and assessment of lymph nodes, including fat dissolution chemicals[6] and ex vivo sentinel lymph node (SLN) identification.[7] With respect to the operative harvesting of nodes, it is recommended to perform a "high tie" of the vascular pedicle to maximize the number of lymph nodes within the colonic mesentery.

WHAT IS THE EVIDENCE TO SUPPORT CURRENT COLONIC CANCER SURGICAL PRACTICE?

It is important to identify the evidence for current practice in colonic cancer surgery. As with most other solid organ malignancies, primary treatment is surgical. In the past, there has been a reluctance to use neoadjuvant therapy in colonic cancer surgery because of concerns over accurate radiological staging and the risk of bowel obstruction during treatment. However, recently published results from the FOxTROT trial show that this option is feasible and safe, and may potentially induce downstaging of disease.[8] In this randomized controlled trial, patients with radiologically staged T3 and T4 colonic tumors were randomized to either preoperative chemotherapy and then surgery or standard postoperative chemotherapy. Early recently reported data indicate low levels of chemotherapy side effects, equivalent levels of postoperative morbidity, and significant downstaging, including 2 reports of pathologic complete response. The trial is now being extended to detect meaningful oncological outcomes at 2 years. Currently there is insufficient evidence to support the routine use of preoperative neoadjuvant chemotherapy in colonic cancer outside of a trial environment.[9]

The tumor must be completely resected; other than isolated case reports in the palliative setting, there is no evidence to support the role of debulking surgery in colon cancer.[10] Because of the high mobility of the colon, resection margins are determined by the degree of lymphovascular dissection required rather than distance from the tumor per se.[11] In general, a distal margin of 5 cm is deemed the minimum necessary, because of the possibility of intramural spread.[2,12,13] There is no evidence to support local resection of colon cancer via colotomies.[2] There is only one randomized trial comparing oncological outcomes in "segmental colectomies" versus hemicolectomies.[14] Segmental colectomy was defined as a localized, not pedicle-based resection of the intestine and this was compared with a traditional pedicle-defined hemicolectomy. In this prospective trial, survival rates were equivalent between patients with left-sided cancers treated with segmental colectomy compared with hemicolectomy. Interestingly, other contemporary retrospective studies have replicated these findings, demonstrating equivalent outcomes comparing segmental colectomies and hemicolectomies for left-sided cancers.[15,16] These isolated data should be interpreted with caution, and on a background of understanding the importance of lymphadenectomy and patterns of lymph node spread. Recent data reinforcing current practice for wide lymphadenectomy and therefore hemicolectomy demonstrates that early lymphatic spread occurs far wider than the juxtatumoral lymph nodes.[17]

The original data suggesting the importance of removing potentially involved lymph nodes was published by Gilchrist and David in 1938.[18] It has since been shown that in stage II and stage III disease, high lymph node yield is positively correlated with survival.[19,20] Interestingly, this study also showed that irrespective of involvement or not, the number of lymph nodes *analyzed* was an independent predictor of outcome even in node-negative cases. The investigators of this study concluded that the surgeon alone may be an important controlling variable. These data and similar studies were reviewed in 2007 by Chang and colleagues,[21] who made broadly similar conclusions. The association of outcome with lymph nodes has been further dissected to reveal a deeper association with that of the ratio of metastatic to total number of identified lymph nodes.[22] Analysis revealed that lymph node *ratio* was a determining factor for overall survival, disease-free survival, and cancer-specific survival if more than 10 lymph nodes were removed. These and many other studies have been used to justify the use of lymph node yield as a surgical end point and surgical quality indicator. As discussed, this is generally held to be important to adequately stage the tumor, thereby preventing understaging, although this direct causation has never been formally shown. From several large studies it is proposed that a minimum of 12 lymph nodes need to be examined to accurately stage the cancer.[23] To acquire and examine adequate numbers of lymph nodes, a complete lymphovascular pedicle is removed en bloc with the specimen. These arterially defined pedicles guide the colonic resection margins to enable restoration of intestinal continuity by anastomosis.

HOW CAN WE IMPROVE ONCOLOGICAL OUTCOMES IN COLON CANCER SURGERY?

Despite some regional differences,[24] over the past 4 decades oncological outcomes for patients with colonic cancer have significantly improved (CRUK Cancer Stats). These have occurred on a background of earlier diagnosis and improvements in adjuvant treatment. However, despite good surgical practice, large numbers of patients with potentially curable colon cancer present with local or distant recurrence following stage I and stage II resections.[25] It has been suggested that circulating tumor cells, micrometastases, and tumor cells residing in immune-privileged areas, such as distinct areas of the bone marrow, may account for some of the unexpected recurrences; it is also possible that surgical practice could be improved.[26] The fundamental issue is whether more aggressive resection might result in more accurate staging, and better oncological outcomes. The newly described technique of complete mesocolic excision (CME) with central vascular ligation (CVL) provides this advantage. The CME approach, from a lymph node retrieval perspective per se, is no different from what is currently done with a "high-tie."

SLN biopsy is used routinely in breast cancer and melanoma surgery. The guiding principle in the technique is that lymph node spread is a marker of systemic disease (Cady-Fisher) and that sensitivity can be improved by sampling solely the first node that a tumor may spread to: the SLN. Should this node be found positive for metastases, adjuvant treatment is necessary. Several studies have attempted to identify whether SLN biopsy can improve identification of lymphatic spread in colorectal cancer above what is currently being performed. The identification of the node is performed in vivo or ex vivo by injecting blue dye, technetium-labeled colloid (99mTc), or indocyanine green fluorescent dye[27] into the normal adjacent bowel. The results from SLN identification in colorectal cancer have been mixed. Two recent systematic reviews of the technique have suggested that the technique may improve staging at the expense of increased workload for either surgeon or pathologist.[7,28]

Experimental approaches to improve staging include serum sampling either before or after surgery to quantify circulating tumor cells (CTC) or tumor DNA and intraoperative bone marrow sampling. There is evidence to support the relationship of both CTCs and bone marrow tumor cells with outcome in colorectal cancer, but reliable and sensitive methodology is not currently available.[26] Identification of circulating tumor DNA may be more promising; it is reported to have greater sensitivity and, by offering individualized mutational analysis, this technique may facilitate targeted adjuvant therapy.

CME AND CVL: BACKGROUND AND SUPPORTIVE EVIDENCE

Rectal cancer surgery was revolutionized by the work of Bill Heald, who reported in 1986 that local recurrence rates could be vastly improved by using the technique of TME.[1] This technique not only removes the primary rectal cancer with an adequate circumferential resection margin, but also removes the mesorectum. The technique of TME improved local recurrence rates from 30% to 40% to as low as 3.7% and is now regarded as the "gold standard" in rectal cancer surgery.

Based on the TME experience, the group from Erlangen in Germany have advocated for CME in conjunction with CVL for colon cancer.[29] CME is reported to differ from traditional colon cancer surgery by achieving a far more radical excision of the lymphovascular pedicle and mesocolon. In addition, the CME technique promotes resection of the specimen with an intact visceral peritoneum together with proximal and distal resection margins of at least 10 cm. Arterial supply to the affected segment of bowel is taken at its origin from the superior mesenteric artery (right and transverse colon) and the aorta (left colon), described as CVL. CME has been shown to lead to increased lymph node harvest and more mesocolic tissue.[30] In a comparison between the Leeds and Erlangen units, it was shown that CME led to an almost doubling in both the number of lymph nodes retrieved and area of mesentery resected. However, a Danish study showed only a 9% increase in lymph node yield.[31]

The Leeds group has since gone on to show that mesocolic *plane* resections alone result in improved 5-year survival outcomes, most apparent in stage III resections.[32] The Erlangen group has also shown that CME improves 5-year survival rates and locoregional recurrence rates for their patients. The improvements are not as marked as with TME, but the improvement in local recurrence, from 6.5% to 3.6%, and in 5-year survival, from 82.1% to 89.1%, are striking.

CME has been shown to be technically feasible in both open and laparoscopic colon surgery.[33] However, a Greek study of 90 patients (41 open and 49 laparoscopic) showed that laparoscopic CME resulted in a marginally shorter distance from tumor to the high tie and slightly fewer lymph nodes in the specimen. An RCT with long-term follow-up remains to be performed to ascertain whether laparoscopic CME can be recommended.

Whether CME is any different from traditional practice in which "high ties" of vascular pedicles are advocated may be debatable.[34] Some of the concepts described in CME are not new; both Enker and colleagues[35] and Turnbull and colleagues[36] stressed the importance of radical lymphadenectomy in improving oncological outcomes.[37] For left-sided tumors, the dissections described by the Erlangen group appear generally similar to traditional descriptions. For right-sided and transverse colon tumors, the Erlangen description involves a much higher tie and dissection, including full mobilization of the duodenum, head of pancreas, and, on occasion, dissection of the gastroepiploic arteries. Interestingly, the reported Erlangen complication rates from their more radical dissections are no different than the traditional approach. Others have identified an increase in genitourinary complications, including ejaculatory dysfunction, with CVL for left-sided tumors.[38] The outcomes of the Erlangen group have since been replicated by others, suggesting that high vascular ligation shows oncological benefit in both local recurrence and 5-year mortality rates.[31] It has also been shown that the practice of CME can be standardized, taught, and implemented with reproducible results.[39]

The apparent improved outcomes with CME are yet to be confirmed with a formal RCT. Proposed explanations for the apparent improvements are that increasing lymph node yield permits stage migration, that increased lymph node yield removes a source of metastases, and that it has nothing to do with lymphatics but is due to the preservation of an intact peritoneum.

WHICH LYMPH NODES DO COLONIC TUMORS SPREAD TO?

The conventional wisdom is that colonic adenocarcinoma spreads to the lymph nodes that are anatomically associated with the arterial supply of the affected colonic segment. Removal of the vascularly defined mesocolon should include all the at-risk lymph nodes distal to the systemic lymphatic channels. Several recent publications have demonstrated that colonic tumors are capable of far wider spread than can be predicted by arterial anatomy. In particular, it appears that right-sided and transverse colon tumors possess highly variable lymphatic spread.[40–42] This can include spread to lymph nodes associated with neighboring vascular pedicles. Although there is significant variation in lymphatic drainage patterns, there is also evidence of variation in arterial supply.[43] Of note is the variable origin and branching patterns of the right and middle colonic arteries. It could be envisaged that with CME advocating a dissection of the vessels to the origin of the superior mesenteric artery for right-sided tumors this may also harvest nonanatomically distributed lymph nodes. At present, the specific lymphatic drainage pattern of individual tumors cannot radiologically or otherwise be identified. This implies that those patients who may benefit from such wider lymphadenectomy cannot reliably be selected. Clearly, if this wider resection is performed uniformly on an unselected population, it may lead to increased morbidity. Identification of which patient or tumor subgroups appear to spread more widely is necessary to enable a more targeted approach to selective wider lymphadenectomy, such as CME.

HOW DOES IMPROVED LYMPH NODE YIELD EQUATE TO IMPROVED SURVIVAL?

It may be prudent to discuss whether the results from CME are a reflection of previous understaging of disease or a direct effect of removal of tumor burden. The concept of en bloc lymph node resection is applicable to almost all other solid organ malignancies. For example, multiple studies have shown in breast cancer that identifying lymph node spread via either SLN biopsy or axillary clearance improves the staging of the disease. It is easy to extrapolate these data to colonic carcinoma, but these are 2 distinct biologic entities and patterns of spread are likely different between them.

Interestingly, a recent observational cohort study looking at US SEER (Surveillance, Epidemiology, and End Results) data that quantified nodal positivity rates, showed that irrespective of surgical technique, this rate remained constant at 40%.[44] Here, Parsons and colleagues also noted that despite increased numbers of lymph nodes retrieved, they did not see an increase in higher-stage tumors. Indeed this 40% value appears to hold even for the radical CME.[29] These fascinating observations suggest that understaging may not be the explanation for apparent improved outcomes and that the explanation may be more complex and possibly biologic. Parsons and colleagues propose that specific tumor growth factors may stimulate lymph node enlargement, which is reflective of an underlying systemic immune response to the tumor, as has also been proposed by others.[45] One important study supporting this hypothesis showed that in an analysis of 843 patients with colon cancer, lymphocytic reaction to the tumor was highly prognostic and independent of total lymph node counts and tumor-specific molecular identifiers, including MSI (microsatellite instability) status, CIMP (CpG island methylator phenotype), and the presence of BRAF mutation.[46] The relevance of this for CME is that the additional lymph nodes retrieved per se may not actually change either prognosis or stage.

A further publication has even shown that the increased lymph node yield achieved with CME, although statistically significant, is not hugely different from that achieved with conventional surgery (26.7 vs 24.5),[31] although the Erlangen and Leeds groups have reported larger differences.[30] It is also very likely that the differences between previous surgical practice and CME are much less pronounced than the differences between TME and pre-TME technique. Indeed, even if the tumor immunology data are ignored, it is questionable whether an increased harvest of a few distant lymph nodes accounts for the improved oncological outcomes shown with CME. What is perhaps more plausible is that the benefit comes from the combination of central vascular ligation together with excision of an intact visceral layer of peritoneum. Little has been written as to the role or importance of transcoelomic spread in colorectal cancer either preoperatively or intraoperatively. However, it is clear that significant numbers of viable cancer cells are present on these peritoneal surfaces and are interestingly correlated with the presence of liver metastases.[47] Solomon and colleagues[47] found that 15% of colorectal cancers had cancer cells on the peritoneal surface of the bowel. From an oncological perspective, it is clear that removal of these potential sources of local and distant recurrence should improve outcomes. It is therefore possible that performing CME removes a greater number of these cells than would be performed using conventional surgery and this may also contribute to the potentially improved oncological effects of CME.

Further complicating and confounding the studies comparing CME and traditional surgery is that generally all the tumors are regarded as being biologically homogeneous. Unlike other tumors, such as breast, where distinct molecular subtypes have been identified,[48] in colorectal cancer the only 2 clinically relevant molecular subtypes are defined by MSI and chromosome instability (CIN) status. Recent publications, however, point to a far more complex and heterogeneous picture more akin to breast cancer where multiple genetically distinct and definable subtypes exist, each with unique behaviors and distinct etiologies.[49,50] It is also highly likely that colorectal cancer is similar in nature to renal cancer, which has recently been shown to possess within individual tumors multiple genetically distinct clones with variable behavior.[51] Complicating this even further are recent data pointing to intratumoral functional heterogeneity within genetically identical cells, where clonal behaviors are additionally defined by epigenetic and microenvironmentally controlled factors.[52] The implications of these multiple layers of heterogeneity are that although a tumor may possess a dominant genetic clone, subclones with different behavior may also exist. Clonal propensity for metastatic spread, be it hematogeneous or lymphatic, are likely highly variable. This emerging complex and dynamic view of colorectal cancer may in time shed light on outcome data comparing traditional lymphadenectomy with CME and the role of lymphadenectomy in general. It is possible that the Cady-Fisher and Halsted theories are not mutually exclusive and that some tumors may require lymphadenectomy to gain surgical control rather than just for staging purposes and vice versa. It will be only through a personalized approach to colorectal cancer treatment with careful molecular classification of the tumor in combination with detailed radiological imaging that will enable targeted surgical treatment; whereas some patients will benefit from CME, some may require only traditional lymphadenectomy, and some may potentially require neither. This latter proposal may be particularly important in light of ongoing technological advances in endoscopic resections that do not assess or remove draining lymph nodes.[53] At the current time, the encouraging results shown with CME need to be confirmed by a formal RCT with long-term follow-up. Until this is demonstrated, the role of CME should be restricted to ethically approved study.

SUMMARY

Apart from the advent of laparoscopic surgery and the newly proposed CME, colonic cancer surgery has changed little over the past few decades. Not least, this must be consequent on an assumption that what is currently performed is the widest oncological resection possible. The improved outcomes demonstrated with CME cannot be completely attributed to stage migration, and this suggests that at least in some patients a more radical surgical approach may be required. CME is a more technically challenging operation, and although the Erlangen experience does not demonstrate increased morbidity, it may not be appropriate or required for all patients with colon cancer. Until patients can be stratified preoperatively into those who may benefit from more extended lymphadenectomy and those who will not, CME should not be routinely adopted.

REFERENCES

1. Heald RJ, Ryall RD. Recurrence and survival after total mesorectal excision for rectal cancer. Lancet 1986;1(8496):1479–82.
2. Chang GJ, Kaiser AM, Mills S, et al. Practice parameters for the management of colon cancer. Dis Colon Rectum 2012;55(8):831–43.
3. Clinical Outcomes of Surgical Therapy Study Group. A comparison of laparoscopically assisted and open colectomy for colon cancer. N Engl J Med 2004; 350(20):2050–9.
4. Green BL, Marshall HC, Collinson F, et al. Long-term follow-up of the Medical Research Council CLASICC trial of conventional versus laparoscopically assisted resection in colorectal cancer. Br J Surg 2013;100(1):75–82.
5. Buunen M, Veldkamp R, Hop WC, et al. Survival after laparoscopic surgery versus open surgery for colon cancer: long-term outcome of a randomised clinical trial. Lancet Oncol 2009;10(1):44–52.
6. Hernanz F, Garcia-Somacarrera E, Fernandez F. The assessment of lymph nodes missed in mesenteric tissue after standard dissection of colorectal cancer specimens. Colorectal Dis 2010;12(7 Online):e57–60.
7. van der Pas MH, Meijer S, Hoekstra OS, et al. Sentinel-lymph-node procedure in colon and rectal cancer: a systematic review and meta-analysis. Lancet Oncol 2011;12(6):540–50.
8. Foxtrot Collaborative Group. Feasibility of preoperative chemotherapy for locally advanced, operable colon cancer: the pilot phase of a randomised controlled trial. Lancet Oncol 2012;13(11):1152–60.
9. Arredondo J, Pastor C, Baixauli J, et al. Preliminary outcome of a treatment strategy based on perioperative chemotherapy and surgery in patients with locally advanced colon cancer. Colorectal Dis 2013;15(5):552–7.
10. Ripley RT, Gajdos C, Reppert AE, et al. Sequential radiofrequency ablation and surgical debulking for unresectable colorectal carcinoma: thermo-surgical ablation. J Surg Oncol 2013;107(2):144–7.
11. Stearns MW Jr, Schottenfeld D. Techniques for the surgical management of colon cancer. Cancer 1971;28(1):165–9.
12. Devereux DF, Deckers PJ. Contributions of pathologic margins and Dukes' stage to local recurrence in colorectal carcinoma. Am J Surg 1985;149(3):323–6.
13. Nelson H, Petrelli N, Carlin A, et al. Guidelines 2000 for colon and rectal cancer surgery. J Natl Cancer Inst 2001;93(8):583–96.
14. Rouffet F, Hay JM, Vacher B, et al. Curative resection for left colonic carcinoma: hemicolectomy vs. segmental colectomy. A prospective, controlled, multicenter trial. French Association for Surgical Research. Dis Colon Rectum 1994;37(7):651–9.
15. Busuttil RW, Foglia RP, Longmire WP Jr. Treatment of carcinoma of the sigmoid colon and upper rectum. A comparison of local segmental resection and left hemicolectomy. Arch Surg 1977;112(8):920–3.
16. Secco GB, Ravera G, Gasparo A, et al. Segmental resection, lymph nodes dissection and survival in patients with left colon cancer. Hepatogastroenterology 2007;54(74):422–6.
17. Tan KY, Kawamura YJ, Mizokami K, et al. Distribution of the first metastatic lymph node in colon cancer and its clinical significance. Colorectal Dis 2010; 12(1):44–7.
18. Gilchrist RK, David VC. Lymphatic spread of carcinoma of the rectum. Ann Surg 1938;108(4):621–42.

19. Le Voyer TE, Sigurdson ER, Hanlon AL, et al. Colon cancer survival is associated with increasing number of lymph nodes analyzed: a secondary survey of intergroup trial INT-0089. J Clin Oncol 2003;21(15):2912–9.

20. Lykke J, Roikjaer O, Jess P. The relation between lymph node status and survival in Stage I-III colon cancer: results from a prospective nationwide cohort study. Colorectal Dis 2013;15(5):559–65.

21. Chang GJ, Rodriguez-Bigas MA, Skibber JM, et al. Lymph node evaluation and survival after curative resection of colon cancer: systematic review. J Natl Cancer Inst 2007;99(6):433–41.

22. Berger AC, Sigurdson ER, LeVoyer T, et al. Colon cancer survival is associated with decreasing ratio of metastatic to examined lymph nodes. J Clin Oncol 2005; 23(34):8706–12.

23. Compton CC, Fielding LP, Burgart LJ, et al. Prognostic factors in colorectal cancer. College of American Pathologists Consensus Statement 1999. Arch Pathol Lab Med 2000;124(7):979–94.

24. Morris EJ, Sandin F, Lambert PC, et al. A population-based comparison of the survival of patients with colorectal cancer in England, Norway and Sweden between 1996 and 2004. Gut 2011;60(8):1087–93.

25. Figueredo A, Coombes ME, Mukherjee S. Adjuvant therapy for completely resected stage II colon cancer. Cochrane Database Syst Rev 2008;(3):CD005390.

26. Rahbari NN, Aigner M, Thorlund K, et al. Meta-analysis shows that detection of circulating tumor cells indicates poor prognosis in patients with colorectal cancer. Gastroenterology 2010;138(5):1714–26.

27. Cahill RA, Anderson M, Wang LM, et al. Near-infrared (NIR) laparoscopy for intraoperative lymphatic road-mapping and sentinel node identification during definitive surgical resection of early-stage colorectal neoplasia. Surg Endosc 2012;26(1):197–204.

28. van der Zaag ES, Bouma WH, Tanis PJ, et al. Systematic review of sentinel lymph node mapping procedure in colorectal cancer. Ann Surg Oncol 2012; 19(11):3449–59.

29. Hohenberger W, Weber K, Matzel K, et al. Standardized surgery for colonic cancer: complete mesocolic excision and central ligation—technical notes and outcome. Colorectal Dis 2009;11(4):354–64 [discussion: 364–5].

30. West NP, Hohenberger W, Weber K, et al. Complete mesocolic excision with central vascular ligation produces an oncologically superior specimen compared with standard surgery for carcinoma of the colon. J Clin Oncol 2010;28(2):272–8.

31. Bertelsen CA, Bols B, Ingeholm P, et al. Can the quality of colonic surgery be improved by standardization of surgical technique with complete mesocolic excision? Colorectal Dis 2011;13(10):1123–9.

32. West NP, Morris EJ, Rotimi O, et al. Pathology grading of colon cancer surgical resection and its association with survival: a retrospective observational study. Lancet Oncol 2008;9(9):857–65.

33. Gouvas N, Pechlivanides G, Zervakis N, et al. Complete mesocolic excision in colon cancer surgery: a comparison between open and laparoscopic approach. Colorectal Dis 2012;14(11):1357–64.

34. Hogan AM, Winter DC. Mesocolic plane surgery: just plain surgery? Colorectal Dis 2009;11(4):430–1.

35. Enker WE, Laffer UT, Block GE. Enhanced survival of patients with colon and rectal cancer is based upon wide anatomic resection. Ann Surg 1979;190(3):350–60.

36. Turnbull RB Jr, Kyle K, Watson FR, et al. Cancer of the colon: the influence of the no-touch isolation technic on survival rates. Ann Surg 1967;166(3):420–7.

37. Bokey EL, Chapuis PH, Dent OF, et al. Surgical technique and survival in patients having a curative resection for colon cancer. Dis Colon Rectum 2003; 46(7):860–6.
38. Liang JT, Huang KC, Lai HS, et al. Oncologic results of laparoscopic D3 lymphadenectomy for male sigmoid and upper rectal cancer with clinically positive lymph nodes. Ann Surg Oncol 2007;14(7):1980–90.
39. West NP, Sutton KM, Ingeholm P, et al. Improving the quality of colon cancer surgery through a surgical education program. Dis Colon Rectum 2010; 53(12):1594–603.
40. Park IJ, Choi GS, Kang BM, et al. Lymph node metastasis patterns in right-sided colon cancers: is segmental resection of these tumors oncologically safe? Ann Surg Oncol 2009;16(6):1501–6.
41. Yada H, Sawai K, Taniguchi H, et al. Analysis of vascular anatomy and lymph node metastases warrants radical segmental bowel resection for colon cancer. World J Surg 1997;21(1):109–15.
42. Toyota S, Ohta H, Anazawa S. Rationale for extent of lymph node dissection for right colon cancer. Dis Colon Rectum 1995;38(7):705–11.
43. Sakorafas GH, Zouros E, Peros G. Applied vascular anatomy of the colon and rectum: clinical implications for the surgical oncologist. Surg Oncol 2006; 15(4):243–55.
44. Parsons HM, Tuttle TM, Kuntz KM, et al. Association between lymph node evaluation for colon cancer and node positivity over the past 20 years. JAMA 2011; 306(10):1089–97.
45. Ogino S, Galon J, Fuchs CS, et al. Cancer immunology—analysis of host and tumor factors for personalized medicine. Nat Rev Clin Oncol 2011;8(12):711–9.
46. Ogino S, Nosho K, Irahara N, et al. Lymphocytic reaction to colorectal cancer is associated with longer survival, independent of lymph node count, microsatellite instability, and CpG island methylator phenotype. Clin Cancer Res 2009;15(20): 6412–20.
47. Solomon MJ, Egan M, Roberts RA, et al. Incidence of free colorectal cancer cells on the peritoneal surface. Dis Colon Rectum 1997;40(11):1294–8.
48. Curtis C, Shah SP, Chin SF, et al. The genomic and transcriptomic architecture of 2,000 breast tumours reveals novel subgroups. Nature 2012;486(7403):346–52.
49. De Sousa EM, Wang X, Jansen M, et al. Poor-prognosis colon cancer is defined by a molecularly distinct subtype and develops from serrated precursor lesions. Nat Med 2013;19(5):614–8.
50. Sadanandam A, Lyssiotis CA, Homicsko K, et al. A colorectal cancer classification system that associates cellular phenotype and responses to therapy. Nat Med 2013;19(5):619–25.
51. Gerlinger M, Rowan AJ, Horswell S, et al. Intratumor heterogeneity and branched evolution revealed by multiregion sequencing. N Engl J Med 2012; 366(10):883–92.
52. Kreso A, O'Brien CA, van Galen P, et al. Variable clonal repopulation dynamics influence chemotherapy response in colorectal cancer. Science 2013; 339(6119):543–8.
53. Brigic A, Symons NR, Faiz O, et al. A systematic review regarding the feasibility and safety of endoscopic full thickness resection (EFTR) for colonic lesions. Surg Endosc 2013;27(10):3520–9.

Controversies in Laparoscopy for Colon and Rectal Cancer

Kellie L. Mathis, MD*, Heidi Nelson, MD

KEYWORDS

- Colon cancer • Rectal cancer • Surgical morbidity • Oncologic outcomes
- Laparoscopic surgery

KEY POINTS

- Laparoscopic surgery should be offered to appropriate patients undergoing colectomy for colon cancer, as oncologic outcomes are equivalent to those following open surgery.
- Laparoscopy for colon cancer offers faster gastrointestinal recovery and shorter duration of hospital stay compared with open surgery.
- Laparoscopic proctectomy for rectal cancer is being studied. Oncologic data are not yet available, but short-term outcomes are at least equivalent to open proctectomy.

INTRODUCTION

Colorectal cancer is the third most common malignancy and the third most common cause of cancer-related death in the United States.[1] Surgical resection remains the primary treatment modality for resectable disease, and the surgical management of colon and rectal cancer has evolved over the past 2 decades. Laparoscopy for colon surgery was originally reported in 1991 by Fowler and White.[2] Since that time, considerable controversy has surrounded the application of laparoscopic techniques for colon and rectal cancer. Despite an abundance of randomized trial evidence that laparoscopy is oncologically equivalent to and offers short-term benefits over open colectomy for colon cancer, laparoscopy remains underused. Early data suggest that short-term benefits are also realized for rectal cancer, but robust long-term oncologic data are not yet available. Laparoscopy in the pelvis is technically challenging and whether laparoscopic proctectomy for rectal cancer is ready for prime time remains to be determined. Robotic rectal dissection may overcome many of the challenges of laparoscopy.

The authors have nothing to disclose.
Division of Colon and Rectal Surgery, Mayo Clinic, 200 First Street Southwest, Rochester, MN 55905, USA
* Corresponding author.
E-mail address: mathis.kellie@mayo.edu

Surg Oncol Clin N Am 23 (2014) 35–47
http://dx.doi.org/10.1016/j.soc.2013.09.006
1055-3207/14/$ – see front matter © 2014 Elsevier Inc. All rights reserved.

It has been suggested that only approximately 9% of colectomies for colon cancer were being performed laparoscopically in the United States between 2005 and 2007.[3] An administrative review of 48 hospitals in the northwest United States showed that there was no increase in the percentage of colon cancer operations performed laparoscopically between 2005 and 2010.[4] Similar findings were reported recently using data from the National Inpatient Sample in which only 6.7% of colon cancer cases were being done laparoscopically.[5] The reasons for this perceived lack of acceptance are not known. Lack of training and/or experience with the technique, as well as persistent concerns about the oncologic adequacy of the technique are likely the 2 major contributing factors. There is also evidence that database reviews underestimate the percentage of patients undergoing laparoscopy for colon cancer. With improved coding, Fox and colleagues[6] reviewed data from the National Inpatient Sample and determined that more than 40% of colon cancer operations are now done laparoscopically. We review the available evidence for the laparoscopic technique for colon and rectal cancer.

COLON CANCER
Operative and Short-Term Outcomes

Level I evidence from 4 large multicenter (often multinational) randomized trials consistently suggest that patients undergoing laparoscopic and open colon cancer surgery have equivalent rates of perioperative morbidity and mortality.[7–10] The operative outcomes and short-term results of these 4 trials are reported in **Tables 1** and **2**.

Multiple meta-analyses and systematic reviews have been performed to combine the short-term outcomes of available randomized controlled trials (RCTs) for laparoscopic versus open colon cancer resection. Tjandra and Chan[11] evaluated 17 randomized trials with a combined 4013 patients. They found no significant differences in overall and surgery-specific morbidity, anastomotic leak rates, reoperation rates, and quality of oncologic resection. Operative times were prolonged in the laparoscopic group. Additionally, laparoscopy was associated with lower 30-day mortality, fewer wound complications, lower surgical blood loss, and decreased pain scores, with an associated lower requirement for narcotic analgesia. Bowel function and

Table 1
Operative outcomes for laparoscopic versus open resection of colon cancer in major randomized trials

Trial	Assigned Group	No. of Patients	Conversion Rate (%)	Operative Time (min)	Estimated Blood Loss (mL)	Lymph Node Count
COST[7]	Laparoscopy	437	21	150	—	12
	Open	435		95	—	12
CLASICC[8]	Laparoscopy	273	29	180	—	12
	Open	140		135	—	14
COLOR I[10]	Laparoscopy	621	17	145	100	10
	Open	627		115	175	10
ALCCaS[9]	Laparoscopy	298	15	158	100	13
	Open	294		107	100	13

Abbreviations: ALCCaS, Australasian Randomized Clinic Study Comparing Laparoscopic and Conventional Open Surgical Treatments for Colon Cancer; CLASICC, Conventional versus Laparoscopic-Assisted Surgery in Colorectal Cancer; COLOR I, Colon Cancer Laparoscopic or Open Resection I; COST, Clinical Outcomes of Surgical Therapy.

Table 2
Short-term outcomes for laparoscopic versus open resection of colon cancer in major randomized trials

Trial	Assigned Group	No. of Patients	Time to 1st BM (d)	Duration of Hospital Stay (d)	30-d Morbidity (%)	30-d or In-Hospital Mortality (%)
COST[7]	Laparoscopy	437	3	5	21	0.5
	Open	435	4	6	20	0.9
CLASICC[8]	Laparoscopy	273	5	9	26	4
	Open	140	6	9	27	5
COLOR I[10]	Laparoscopy	621	3.6	8	21	1
	Open	627	4.6	9	20	2
ALCCaS[9]	Laparoscopy	298	4	10	38	1.4
	Open	294	5	11	45	0.7

Abbreviations: ALCCaS, Australasian Randomized Clinic Study Comparing Laparoscopic and Conventional Open Surgical Treatments for Colon Cancer; BM, Bowel Movement; CLASICC, Conventional versus Laparoscopic-Assisted Surgery in Colorectal Cancer; COLOR I, Colon Cancer Laparoscopic or Open Resection I; COST, Clinical Outcomes of Surgical Therapy.

oral diet were earlier, and duration of hospital stay was shorter by 1.7 days in the laparoscopic group. A Cochrane database review included 25 randomized trials. They found an increased operative time in the laparoscopic group; the open group had higher blood loss, higher pain scores, longer duration of ileus, and longer length of stay. Overall morbidity and surgery-specific morbidity were also improved in the laparoscopic group. Nonsurgical morbidity and mortality were not different.[12] An additional systematic review of 19 trials showed no difference in the number of lymph nodes harvested or in the completeness of surgical resection.[13]

Long-Term Oncologic Outcomes

All 4 of the major randomized trials have reported long-term oncologic outcomes for a minimum of 3 years.[14–17] There were no differences in overall or disease-free survival (**Table 3**).

Bonjer and colleagues[18] confirmed no difference in survival outcomes when the Clinical Outcomes of Surgical Therapy (COST), Colon Cancer Laparoscopic or Open Resection (COLOR I), and Conventional Versus Laparoscopic-Assisted Surgery in Colorectal Cancer (CLASICC) trials were combined in a meta-analysis. Other meta-analyses and systematic reviews have combined data from additional single-institution randomized trials and have come to the same conclusion.[13,19]

One randomized study from Barcelona, Spain, compared 111 patients undergoing laparoscopy for colon cancer with 108 undergoing open colectomy. The investigators found that patients in the laparoscopic group had better oncologic outcomes, including lower recurrence rates and improved overall and cancer-specific survival. The differences in this trial were primarily attributable to patients with stage III disease,[20] and these results were not duplicated in larger RCTs.

A Cochrane review of 12 RCTs (3346 patients) comparing laparoscopic and open resection for colorectal cancer reported that in addition to comparable survival and local recurrence rates between groups, there were no differences in the number of reoperations for hernias or adhesions.[21]

Initial concerns were raised about the possibility of higher numbers of port-site and wound recurrences in laparoscopic resections. Long-term follow-up studies have

Table 3
Long-term oncologic outcomes for laparoscopic versus open resection of colon cancer in major randomized trials

Trial	Assigned Group	No. of Patients	Recurrence (%)	Port-Site Recurrence (%)	Disease-Free Survival (%)	Overall Survival (%)
COST[7,16]	Laparoscopy	437	19[a]	0.9[a]	69[a]	76[a]
	Open	435	22	0.5	68	76
CLASICC[17]	Laparoscopy	273	11[a]	2.4[a]	58[a]	56[a]
	Open	140	9	0.5	64	63
COLOR I[15]	Laparoscopy	621	—	1.3[b]	74[b]	82[b]
	Open	627	—	0.4	76	84
ALCCaS[14]	Laparoscopy	298	14[a]	—	72[a]	78[a]
	Open	294	15	—	72	76

Abbreviations: ALCCaS, Australasian Randomized Clinic Study Comparing Laparoscopic and Conventional Open Surgical Treatments for Colon Cancer; CLASICC, Conventional versus Laparoscopic-Assisted Surgery in Colorectal Cancer; COLOR I, Colon Cancer Laparoscopic or Open Resection I; COST, Clinical Outcomes of Surgical Therapy.
[a] Five-year outcomes.
[b] Three-year outcomes.

shown no difference in the rate of port-site recurrences between patients undergoing laparoscopic and open colon cancer surgery.[19] The rate of port-site recurrence was estimated to be 0.6% in a large retrospective study.[22]

It should be noted that most of the RCTs included surgeons with vast laparoscopic experience in high-volume hospitals. Some of the trials used technical credentialing techniques before surgeon approval to enroll patients. Whether the noncredentialed surgeon can achieve the same results is still debated, but recent literature suggests that the answer is yes. McKay and colleagues[23] described short-term outcomes following laparoscopic versus open surgery for colon and rectal cancers in a population-based study in the western zone of Sydney, Australia. The catchment area encompassed 6 hospitals and 36 surgeons. This was a consecutive, nonrandomized series that included 1938 patients undergoing operations over an 8-year period. Specimen adequacy was similar between the open and laparoscopic groups. Conversion rates were low at 6.5% for colon and 8.3% for rectal resection. There were no differences between the open and laparoscopic groups with regard to anastomotic leak, sepsis, reoperation rates, and 30-day mortality. Duration of hospital stay was 7 days in the laparoscopic group and 10 days in the open group. Overall complication rates were lower in the laparoscopic group (32% vs 57%). This study suggests that the benefits seen in the large randomized trials at specialized centers can be translated to the general population of surgeons who have been adequately trained in laparoscopic colon and rectal surgery.

To summarize, data from randomized trials and from single institutions confirms the safety and oncologic adequacy of laparoscopic surgery for the treatment of colon cancer. In view of the easier and faster recovery, laparoscopic resection should be the preferred approach for colon cancer.

RECTAL CANCER
Short-Term Outcomes

The CLASICC trial also included patients with rectal cancer. The investigators found no differences in short-term morbidity or mortality, and the laparoscopic group had a shorter length of hospital stay (by 2 days). Positive circumferential radial margins (CRMs) occurred in 12% of the laparoscopic anterior resection group versus 6% of the open group; for abdominoperineal resections, positive CRMs occurred in 20% of the laparoscopic group and 26% of the open group. The conversion rate to open surgery was high at 34%.[8,24] It should be noted that preoperative pelvic imaging was not routinely performed in this trial, and this may have influenced the conversion rate.

The European COLOR II trial recently reported their short-term outcomes. The trial was performed at 30 hospitals across 8 countries between 2004 and 2010. A total of 1103 patients were randomized to laparoscopic (n = 739) or open surgery (n = 364). No significant differences were seen in completeness of resection, positive CRM rates, morbidity, or mortality. The laparoscopic group experienced lower blood loss, longer operative times, faster return of bowel function, and shorter length of stay.[25] The oncologic results are pending and will likely be reported in the next 2 years.

Systematic reviews and meta-analyses have shown advantages for the laparoscopic groups with regard to wound infection rates, overall morbidity, and length of stay.[26–28] Aziz and colleagues[26] found no difference in CRM positivity between the laparoscopic and open groups. Multiple authors have reported no difference in lymph node counts when comparing laparoscopic and open rectal cancer resection.[29–32]

The American College of Surgeons National Surgical Quality Improvement Program (NSQIP) study evaluated 5240 patients undergoing proctectomy for rectal cancer (19.2% were performed laparoscopically and the remainder were performed open). Laparoscopy resulted in fewer blood transfusions, longer operative times, shorter length of hospital stay (by 2 days), and less morbidity (21% vs 29%). Obese patients had more complications in both groups.[33]

The largest single-institution retrospective review of 579 patients undergoing laparoscopic proctectomy for cancer showed a CRM positivity rate of 2%.[30] Two randomized trials comparing laparoscopic and open proctectomy have found CRM positivity rates of 2.6% to 4.0% in the laparoscopic arms.[34,35] Others have reported a more complete mesorectal fascia following laparoscopic total mesorectal excision (TME) than those undergoing open TME.[36]

Tables 4 and **5** summarize the short-term and operative outcomes for the major randomized trials and meta-analyses.

Table 4
Operative outcomes for laparoscopic versus open resection of rectal cancer in major randomized trials and meta-analyses

Trial	Assigned Group	No. of Patients	Conversion Rate (%)	Operative Time (min)	Estimated Blood Loss (mL)	Lymph Node Count (mean)	Positive CRM Rate (%)
COLOR II[25]	Laparoscopy	739	17	240	200	13	10
	Open	364		188	400	14	10
CLASICC[8]	Laparoscopy	230	34	180	—	8	16
	Open	113		135	—	7	14
Meta-analyses							
Arezzo[71]	Laparoscopy	2087	13	219	307	—	—
	Open	2452		175	444	—	—

Abbreviations: CLASICC, Conventional versus Laparoscopic-Assisted Surgery in Colorectal Cancer; COLOR II, Colon Cancer Laparoscopic or Open Resection II; CRM, circumferential radial margins.

Table 5
Short-term outcomes for laparoscopic versus open resection of rectal cancer in major randomized trials and meta-analyses

Trial	Assigned Group	No. of Patients	Time to GI Function (d)	Duration of Hospital Stay (d)	Morbidity (%)	Mortality (%)	Anastomotic Leak Rate (%)
COLOR II[25]	Laparoscopy	739	2	8	40	1	13
	Open	364	3	9	37	2	10
CLASICC[8]	Laparoscopy	230	5	11	37	4	10
	Open	113	6	13	40	5	7
Meta-analyses							
Arezzo[71]	Laparoscopy	2087	3	11	32	1	8
	Open	2452	4	14	35	4	9

Abbreviations: CLASICC, Conventional versus Laparoscopic-Assisted Surgery in Colorectal Cancer; COLOR II, Colon Cancer Laparoscopic or Open Resection II; GI, gastrointestinal.

Long-Term Outcomes

Data are limited regarding the oncologic outcomes following laparoscopic rectal cancer surgery. In the CLASICC trial, 5-year oncologic overall and disease-free survival outcomes in 381 patients with rectal cancer were not different. Local and distant recurrence rates were also comparable.[17]

The meta-analysis by Aziz and colleagues[26] found no difference in oncologic outcomes between open and laparoscopic TME. Ng and colleagues[34] described no difference in outcomes at 10 years. Other randomized multicenter trials are ongoing, including the COLOR II,[37] the Comparison of Open versus laparoscopic surgery for mid and low REctal cancer After Neoadjuvant chemoradiotherapy (COREAN) trial,[38] Japan Clinical Oncology Group Study (JCOG) 0404,[39] the Australasian Laparoscopic Cancer of the Rectum Trial, and the American College of Surgeons Oncology Group Z6051 trial. **Table 6** reviews the oncologic outcomes available in the reported trials.

CONVERSION RATES

As mentioned earlier, the conversion rate in the CLASICC trial was 34% for laparoscopic rectal cancer surgery.[8] In a 10-year randomized single-institution study comparing laparoscopic and open rectal cancer surgery, the overall conversion rate was 30%.[30] More-recent studies have reported conversion rates that are much lower, ranging from 5% to 8%.[23,40,41] Factors shown to be associated with conversion are high body mass index (BMI), male sex, and locally advanced tumors.[42]

Table 6
Oncologic outcomes for laparoscopic versus open resection of rectal cancer in major randomized trials

Trial	Assigned Group	No. of Patients	Local Recurrence (%)	Disease-Free Survival (%)	Overall Survival (%)
CLASICC[17]	Laparoscopy	230	9–18[a]	53[a]	60[a]
	Open	113	9–18	52	53

Abbreviation: CLASICC, Conventional versus Laparoscopic-Assisted Surgery in Colorectal Cancer.
[a] Five-year outcomes.

At least one study found that patients who require conversion during laparoscopic TME experience inferior oncologic outcomes. It is not clear if this decrease in survival is due to the conversion itself or the factors that precipitated conversion. CLASICC investigators found a significantly lower overall survival at 5 years in patients requiring conversion, but there was no difference in disease-free survival between laparoscopic and converted patients.[17] Similar results were reported in a 10-year retrospective single-institution review of laparoscopic rectal cancer surgery.[43]

LYMPH NODE HARVEST

A meta-analysis of all randomized trials of laparoscopic versus open colorectal cancer surgery (24 studies and 6264 patients) found no difference in the total lymph node count. Lymph node counts were also equivalent when colon cancers and rectal cancers were analyzed separately.[44] Similar findings were shown in another meta-analysis.[45]

COST-EFFECTIVENESS OF LAPAROSCOPY

Jensen and colleagues[46] were the first to study both cost and quality of life in a cost-effectiveness model using data from the randomized trials and meta-analyses. They found that laparoscopic resection for colorectal cancer resulted in a net savings of $4283 per patient with no difference in quality-adjusted life years. Therefore, they consider laparoscopy to be a "dominant strategy" because it results in a cost savings and remains equivalent in quality. Multiple sensitivity analyses produced the same conclusion. A Cochrane systematic review of 48 studies (4224 patients) showed that laparoscopic TME resulted in higher cost.[28]

OBESITY AND LAPAROSCOPY

There are few studies examining the effects of obesity on laparoscopic outcomes for patients with cancer. A Danish study compared short-term outcomes between 93 patients with a BMI of 30 or higher and 332 patients with a BMI lower than 30 undergoing laparoscopic surgery for colorectal cancer. The investigators found no difference in surgical and nonsurgical complication rates, reoperation rates, return of bowel function, or duration of hospital stay. The obese group had significantly longer operative times and increased blood loss. The conversion rate was 29% in the obese group versus 21% in the nonobese group, but this difference was not statistically significant.[47] Makino and colleagues[48] studied the impact of obesity on perioperative outcomes for colorectal laparoscopic operations in a comprehensive review of 33 studies. They found longer operative times and higher conversion rates (in 5 studies) but no other significant differences in morbidity in most of the studies (4 studies did show increased morbidity).

Limited data exist regarding oncologic outcomes between obese and nonobese patients undergoing laparoscopy for colorectal cancer. Singh and colleagues[49] found no differences in overall or disease-free survival at 2 years between obese and nonobese patients. The conversion rate for laparoscopic proctectomy in obese patients was high at 44%.

LAPAROSCOPY IN THE ELDERLY PATIENT

The benefits of laparoscopy may be greatest in the elderly. Stocchi and colleagues[50] found lower rates of morbidity, less narcotic use, shorter length of stay, and shorter postoperative ileus in patients older than 75 years undergoing laparoscopic colectomy when compared with patients undergoing open surgery in a case-matched retrospective review. Additionally, postoperative independence was higher in the laparoscopy group. Advantages in short-term outcomes in elderly patients have also been shown by other investigators.[51–54] In a nonrandomized comparison of rectosigmoid resection in patients older than 70 years, 5-year overall survival was improved in patients undergoing laparoscopic versus open resection.[55]

PELVIC NERVES

TME is associated with a risk of erectile and bladder dysfunction. Kim and colleagues[56] studied the risk prospectively in 68 men undergoing open TME and found that 6% of patients could not successfully obtain/maintain an erection and 13% experienced retrograde ejaculation postoperatively. Sexual desire and satisfaction were decreased in 57% and 63% of patients, respectively. It is unclear how the laparoscopic approach will affect genitourinary function. Stamopoulos and colleagues[57] prospectively measured sexual function before and after treatment for rectal cancer. Fifty-six patients underwent proctectomy (38 open, 18 laparoscopic) and there were significant reductions in International Index of Erectile Function scores in the entire group postoperatively. There were no significant differences between the laparoscopic and open groups at 3 or 6 months. Another prospective study measured voiding and sexual function following laparoscopic and robotic TME in 69 patients. No significant differences were found between the 2 groups.[58]

Results from the CLASICC study showed no difference in bladder function between the laparoscopic and open groups undergoing TME. There was no statistically significant difference in erectile function between groups, but there was a trend toward worse sexual function in the patients undergoing laparoscopic resection.[59]

LEARNING CURVE FOR LAPAROSCOPY

Laparoscopic colorectal surgery is technically challenging, and evidence suggests that there is a steep learning curve. The COST and CLASICC trials required a minimum of 20 laparoscopic colectomies for benign disease as well as a video submission of a laparoscopic segmental colectomy before technical credentialing for trial participation. Random video audits were also performed throughout the trials.[7,8] But most investigators suggest that more resections are necessary before achieving better outcomes. Schlachta and colleagues[60] found that after 30 laparoscopic colectomies, operative times, intraoperative complication rates, and the need for conversion to open surgery all decreased. Others have described learning curves of 55 for right colectomy and 62 for left colectomy.[61] Son and colleagues[62] found that for a single surgeon doing laparoscopic TME, operative time and that the postoperative complication rate stabilized after case number 79. Other studies suggest that the learning curve is even longer for TME (>120 cases) when considering oncologic outcomes, such as local recurrence.[63]

The American Society of Colon and Rectal Surgeons originally prohibited surgeons from performing laparoscopic TME outside of the clinical trial setting, but the most recent practice parameters state that laparoscopic and open TME have equivalent oncologic outcomes and that experienced laparoscopic surgeons who have the technical expertise to perform this procedure can do so within the setting of a clinical trial or an audit that includes long-term outcomes.[64]

Mentoring and telementoring for laparoscopic colon surgery have been described.[65] There are obvious concerns about medical liability, hospital privileges, and compensation that have to be addressed before this can be adopted widely.

SINGLE-INCISION LAPAROSCOPIC COLECTOMY

There are few robust data on outcomes following single-incision laparoscopic colectomy (SILC) for cancer. Single-incision surgery is technically challenging because of the decreased freedom of motion for the surgeon and for the assistant running the camera and the necessity of cross-hand operating. Kim and colleagues[66] compared short-term outcomes between conventional multiport laparoscopy and SILC for colorectal cancer in 179 patients. Margin status and lymph node counts were not different. Postoperative return of bowel function and length of stay were both faster in the SILC group. A systematic review of SILC for colectomy (13 total studies, not all done for cancers) reported low morbidity (13%) and mortality (0.5%). Only 2 studies showed that duration of hospital stay was shorter with SILC than with hand-assisted laparoscopic or conventional multiport laparoscopic colectomy.[67]

ROBOTIC SURGERY FOR RECTAL CANCER

There is a steep learning curve for laparoscopic proctectomy, which is partly due to the limitations of the instruments, the 2-dimensional (2D) visualization with standard laparoscopy, and the difficulty with retraction and exposure in the pelvis. Robotic surgery offers several advantages, such as 3D visualization, a surgeon-controlled camera and additional instrument, endo-wristed instruments, and fixed third-arm retraction. Whether these potential advantages will translate into improvement in outcomes remains to be determined.

A nonrandomized comparison of open versus robotic TME in 82 patients (robotic in 36, laparoscopic mobilization of the colon followed by open TME through a hand port in 46) has been reported. Operative time was longer in the robotic group, but this group had less blood loss. There was no significant difference in the rate of postoperative complications. No patients in the robotic group had a positive CRM versus 3 patients in the open group (P = nonsignificant).[68]

Randomized comparisons between laparoscopic and robotic proctectomy have been described. Baik and colleagues[69] randomized 113 patients; the conversion rate to open surgery was 0% in the robotic group and 11% in the laparoscopy group. The major complication rate was lower in the robotic group (5% vs 19%), and mesorectal grade was superior in the robotic group.

A nonrandomized comparison of laparoscopic versus robotic versus open TME has been reported in 263 patients with rectal cancer. The investigators found no significant differences in specimen quality (judged by distal margin length, lymph node count, and CRM positivity rate) or in complication rates among the 3 groups. The laparoscopic and robotic groups had significantly faster recovery than those in the open group. There was no improvement in short-term outcomes in the robotic cases compared with the laparoscopic cases.[70]

SUMMARY

There is sufficient level I evidence to support and even recommend laparoscopy as the surgical modality of choice for colectomy for colon cancer. Laparoscopy offers improved short-term outcomes and at least equivalent long-term oncologic outcomes when compared to the standard open resection.

Laparoscopic rectal cancer surgery remains investigational. Short-term results from a large multinational randomized trial have just been released and suggest that laparoscopy is not inferior to open total mesorectal excision with regard to completeness of resection and short term morbidity and mortality. Further study is ongoing and it is necessary to await the long-term oncologic results before embracing laparoscopic proctectomy for rectal cancer.

REFERENCES

1. Siegel R, Naishadham D, Jemal A. Cancer statistics, 2013. CA Cancer J Clin 2013;63(1):11–30.
2. Fowler DL, White SA. Laparoscopy-assisted sigmoid resection. Surg Laparosc Endosc 1991;1(3):183–8.
3. Rea JD, Cone MM, Diggs BS, et al. Utilization of laparoscopic colectomy in the United States before and after the clinical outcomes of surgical therapy study group trial. Ann Surg 2011;254(2):281–8.
4. Kwon S, Billingham R, Farrokhi E, et al. Adoption of laparoscopy for elective colorectal resection: a report from the Surgical Care and Outcomes Assessment Program. J Am Coll Surg 2012;214(6):909–18.e1.
5. Robinson CN, Chen GJ, Balentine CJ, et al. Minimally invasive surgery is underutilized for colon cancer. Ann Surg Oncol 2011;18(5):1412–8.
6. Fox J, Gross CP, Longo W, et al. Laparoscopic colectomy for the treatment of cancer has been widely adopted in the United States. Dis Colon Rectum 2012;55(5): 501–8.
7. Clinical Outcomes of Surgical Therapy Study Group. A comparison of laparoscopically assisted and open colectomy for colon cancer. N Engl J Med 2004; 350(20):2050–9.
8. Guillou PJ, Quirke P, Thorpe H, et al. Short-term endpoints of conventional versus laparoscopic-assisted surgery in patients with colorectal cancer (MRC CLASICC trial): multicentre, randomised controlled trial. Lancet 2005;365(9472):1718–26.
9. Hewett PJ, Allardyce RA, Bagshaw PF, et al. Short-term outcomes of the Australasian randomized clinical study comparing laparoscopic and conventional open surgical treatments for colon cancer: the ALCCaS trial. Ann Surg 2008; 248(5):728–38.
10. Veldkamp R, Kuhry E, Hop WC, et al. Laparoscopic surgery versus open surgery for colon cancer: short-term outcomes of a randomised trial. Lancet Oncol 2005;6(7):477–84.
11. Tjandra JJ, Chan MK. Systematic review on the short-term outcome of laparoscopic resection for colon and rectosigmoid cancer. Colorectal Dis 2006;8(5): 375–88.
12. Schwenk W, Haase O, Neudecker J, et al. Short term benefits for laparoscopic colorectal resection. Cochrane Database Syst Rev 2005;(3):CD003145.
13. Lourenco T, Murray A, Grant A, et al. Laparoscopic surgery for colorectal cancer: safe and effective? A systematic review. Surg Endosc 2008;22(5):1146–60.
14. Bagshaw PF, Allardyce RA, Frampton CM, et al. Long-term outcomes of the Australasian randomized clinical trial comparing laparoscopic and conventional open surgical treatments for colon cancer: the Australasian Laparoscopic Colon Cancer Study trial. Ann Surg 2012;256(6):915–9.
15. Buunen M, Veldkamp R, Hop WC, et al. Survival after laparoscopic surgery versus open surgery for colon cancer: long-term outcome of a randomised clinical trial. Lancet Oncol 2009;10(1):44–52.
16. Fleshman J, Sargent DJ, Green E, et al. Laparoscopic colectomy for cancer is not inferior to open surgery based on 5-year data from the COST Study Group trial. Ann Surg 2007;246(4):655–62 [discussion: 662–4].

17. Jayne DG, Thorpe HC, Copeland J, et al. Five-year follow-up of the Medical Research Council CLASICC trial of laparoscopically assisted versus open surgery for colorectal cancer. Br J Surg 2010;97(11):1638–45.

18. Bonjer HJ, Hop WC, Nelson H, et al. Laparoscopically assisted vs open colectomy for colon cancer: a meta-analysis. Arch Surg 2007;142(3):298–303.

19. Jackson TD, Kaplan GG, Arena G, et al. Laparoscopic versus open resection for colorectal cancer: a metaanalysis of oncologic outcomes. J Am Coll Surg 2007; 204(3):439–46.

20. Lacy AM, Garcia-Valdecasas JC, Delgado S, et al. Laparoscopy-assisted colectomy versus open colectomy for treatment of non-metastatic colon cancer: a randomised trial. Lancet 2002;359(9325):2224–9.

21. Kuhry E, Schwenk WF, Gaupset R, et al. Long-term results of laparoscopic colorectal cancer resection. Cochrane Database Syst Rev 2008;(2):CD003432.

22. Reilly WT, Nelson H, Schroeder G, et al. Wound recurrence following conventional treatment of colorectal cancer. A rare but perhaps underestimated problem. Dis Colon Rectum 1996;39(2):200–7.

23. McKay GD, Morgan MJ, Wong SK, et al. Improved short-term outcomes of laparoscopic versus open resection for colon and rectal cancer in an area health service: a multicenter study. Dis Colon Rectum 2012;55(1):42–50.

24. Jayne DG, Guillou PJ, Thorpe H, et al. Randomized trial of laparoscopic-assisted resection of colorectal carcinoma: 3-year results of the UK MRC CLASICC Trial Group. J Clin Oncol 2007;25(21):3061–8.

25. van der Pas MH, Haglind E, Cuesta MA, et al. Laparoscopic versus open surgery for rectal cancer (COLOR II): short-term outcomes of a randomised, phase 3 trial. Lancet Oncol 2013;14(3):210–8.

26. Aziz O, Constantinides V, Tekkis PP, et al. Laparoscopic versus open surgery for rectal cancer: a meta-analysis. Ann Surg Oncol 2006;13(3):413–24.

27. Gao F, Cao YF, Chen LS. Meta-analysis of short-term outcomes after laparoscopic resection for rectal cancer. Int J Colorectal Dis 2006;21(7):652–6.

28. Breukink S, Pierie J, Wiggers T. Laparoscopic versus open total mesorectal excision for rectal cancer. Cochrane Database Syst Rev 2006;(4):CD005200.

29. Braga M, Frasson M, Vignali A, et al. Laparoscopic resection in rectal cancer patients: outcome and cost-benefit analysis. Dis Colon Rectum 2007;50(4): 464–71.

30. Ng KH, Ng DC, Cheung HY, et al. Laparoscopic resection for rectal cancers: lessons learned from 579 cases. Ann Surg 2009;249(1):82–6.

31. Bretagnol F, Lelong B, Laurent C, et al. The oncological safety of laparoscopic total mesorectal excision with sphincter preservation for rectal carcinoma. Surg Endosc 2005;19(7):892–6.

32. Law WL, Lee YM, Choi HK, et al. Laparoscopic and open anterior resection for upper and mid rectal cancer: an evaluation of outcomes. Dis Colon Rectum 2006;49(8):1108–15.

33. Greenblatt DY, Rajamanickam V, Pugely AJ, et al. Short-term outcomes after laparoscopic-assisted proctectomy for rectal cancer: results from the ACS NSQIP. J Am Coll Surg 2011;212(5):844–54.

34. Ng SS, Leung KL, Lee JF, et al. Long-term morbidity and oncologic outcomes of laparoscopic-assisted anterior resection for upper rectal cancer: ten-year results of a prospective, randomized trial. Dis Colon Rectum 2009;52(4):558–66.

35. Lujan J, Valero G, Hernandez Q, et al. Randomized clinical trial comparing laparoscopic and open surgery in patients with rectal cancer. Br J Surg 2009;96(9): 982–9.

36. Gouvas N, Tsiaoussis J, Pechlivanides G, et al. Quality of surgery for rectal car-cinoma: comparison between open and laparoscopic approaches. Am J Surg 2009;198(5):702–8.
37. Buunen M, Bonjer HJ, Hop WC, et al. COLOR II. A randomized clinical trial comparing laparoscopic and open surgery for rectal cancer. Dan Med Bull 2009;56(2):89–91.
38. Kang SB, Park JW, Jeong SY, et al. Open versus laparoscopic surgery for mid or low rectal cancer after neoadjuvant chemoradiotherapy (COREAN trial): short-term outcomes of an open-label randomised controlled trial. Lancet Oncol 2010;11(7):637–45.
39. Kitano S, Inomata M, Sato A, et al. Randomized controlled trial to evaluate lapa-roscopic surgery for colorectal cancer: Japan Clinical Oncology Group Study JCOG 0404. Jpn J Clin Oncol 2005;35(8):475–7.
40. Miyajima N, Fukunaga M, Hasegawa H, et al. Results of a multicenter study of 1,057 cases of rectal cancer treated by laparoscopic surgery. Surg Endosc 2009;23(1):113–8.
41. Bege T, Lelong B, Esterni B, et al. The learning curve for the laparoscopic approach to conservative mesorectal excision for rectal cancer: lessons drawn from a single institution's experience. Ann Surg 2010;251(2):249–53.
42. Thorpe H, Jayne DG, Guillou PJ, et al. Patient factors influencing conversion from laparoscopically assisted to open surgery for colorectal cancer. Br J Surg 2008;95(2):199–205.
43. Rottoli M, Bona S, Rosati R, et al. Laparoscopic rectal resection for cancer: effects of conversion on short-term outcome and survival. Ann Surg Oncol 2009;16(5):1279–86.
44. Wu Z, Zhang S, Aung LH, et al. Lymph node harvested in laparoscopic versus open colorectal cancer approaches: a meta-analysis. Surg Laparosc Endosc Percutan Tech 2012;22(1):5–11.
45. Abraham NS, Young JM, Solomon MJ. Meta-analysis of short-term outcomes af-ter laparoscopic resection for colorectal cancer. Br J Surg 2004;91(9):1111–24.
46. Jensen CC, Prasad LM, Abcarian H. Cost-effectiveness of laparoscopic vs open resection for colon and rectal cancer. Dis Colon Rectum 2012;55(10):1017–23.
47. Poulsen M, Ovesen H. Is laparoscopic colorectal cancer surgery in obese pa-tients associated with an increased risk? Short-term results from a single center study of 425 patients. J Gastrointest Surg 2012;16(8):1554–8.
48. Makino T, Shukla PJ, Rubino F, et al. The impact of obesity on perioperative out-comes after laparoscopic colorectal resection. Ann Surg 2012;255(2):228–36.
49. Singh A, Muthukumarasamy G, Pawa N, et al. Laparoscopic colorectal cancer surgery in obese patients. Colorectal Dis 2011;13(8):878–83.
50. Stocchi L, Nelson H, Young-Fadok TM, et al. Safety and advantages of laparo-scopic vs. open colectomy in the elderly: matched-control study. Dis Colon Rectum 2000;43(3):326–32.
51. Law WL, Chu KW, Tung PH. Laparoscopic colorectal resection: a safe option for elderly patients. J Am Coll Surg 2002;195(6):768–73.
52. Tuech JJ, Pessaux P, Rouge C, et al. Laparoscopic vs open colectomy for sig-moid diverticulitis: a prospective comparative study in the elderly. Surg Endosc 2000;14(11):1031–3.
53. Frasson M, Braga M, Vignali A, et al. Benefits of laparoscopic colorectal resection are more pronounced in elderly patients. Dis Colon Rectum 2008;51(3):296–300.
54. Senagore AJ, Madbouly KM, Fazio VW, et al. Advantages of laparoscopic colec-tomy in older patients. Arch Surg 2003;138(3):252–6.

55. Altuntas YE, Gezen C, Vural S, et al. Laparoscopy for sigmoid colon and rectal cancers in septuagenarians: a retrospective, comparative study. Tech Coloproctol 2012;16(3):213–9.

56. Kim NK, Aahn TW, Park JK, et al. Assessment of sexual and voiding function after total mesorectal excision with pelvic autonomic nerve preservation in males with rectal cancer. Dis Colon Rectum 2002;45(9):1178–85.

57. Stamopoulos P, Theodoropoulos GE, Papailiou J, et al. Prospective evaluation of sexual function after open and laparoscopic surgery for rectal cancer. Surg Endosc 2009;23(12):2665–74.

58. Kim JY, Kim NK, Lee KY, et al. A comparative study of voiding and sexual function after total mesorectal excision with autonomic nerve preservation for rectal cancer: laparoscopic versus robotic surgery. Ann Surg Oncol 2012;19(8): 2485–93.

59. Jayne DG, Brown JM, Thorpe H, et al. Bladder and sexual function following resection for rectal cancer in a randomized clinical trial of laparoscopic versus open technique. Br J Surg 2005;92(9):1124–32.

60. Schlachta CM, Mamazza J, Seshadri PA, et al. Defining a learning curve for laparoscopic colorectal resections. Dis Colon Rectum 2001;44(2):217–22.

61. Tekkis PP, Senagore AJ, Delaney CP, et al. Evaluation of the learning curve in laparoscopic colorectal surgery: comparison of right-sided and left-sided resections. Ann Surg 2005;242(1):83–91.

62. Son GM, Kim JG, Lee JC, et al. Multidimensional analysis of the learning curve for laparoscopic rectal cancer surgery. J Laparoendosc Adv Surg Tech A 2010; 20(7):609–17.

63. Park IJ, Choi GS, Lim KH, et al. Multidimensional analysis of the learning curve for laparoscopic resection in rectal cancer. J Gastrointest Surg 2009;13(2): 275–81.

64. Monson JR, Weiser MR, Buie WD, et al. Practice parameters for the management of rectal cancer (revised). Dis Colon Rectum 2013;56(5):535–50.

65. Schlachta CM, Sorsdahl AK, Lefebvre KL, et al. A model for longitudinal mentoring and telementoring of laparoscopic colon surgery. Surg Endosc 2009;23(7): 1634–8.

66. Kim SJ, Ryu GO, Choi BJ, et al. The short-term outcomes of conventional and single-port laparoscopic surgery for colorectal cancer. Ann Surg 2011;254(6): 933–40.

67. Makino T, Milsom JW, Lee SW. Feasibility and safety of single-incision laparoscopic colectomy: a systematic review. Ann Surg 2012;255(4):667–76.

68. deSouza AL, Prasad LM, Ricci J, et al. A comparison of open and robotic total mesorectal excision for rectal adenocarcinoma. Dis Colon Rectum 2011;54(3): 275–82.

69. Baik SH, Kwon HY, Kim JS, et al. Robotic versus laparoscopic low anterior resection of rectal cancer: short-term outcome of a prospective comparative study. Ann Surg Oncol 2009;16(6):1480–7.

70. Park JS, Choi GS, Lim KH, et al. S052: a comparison of robot-assisted, laparoscopic, and open surgery in the treatment of rectal cancer. Surg Endosc 2011; 25(1):240–8.

71. Arezzo A, Passera R, Scozzari G, et al. Laparoscopy for rectal cancer reduces short-term mortality and morbidity: results of a systematic review and meta-analysis. Surg Endosc 2013;27(5):1485–502.

Current Practices and Challenges of Adjuvant Chemotherapy in Patients with Colorectal Cancer

Christine Brezden-Masley, MD, PhD, FRCPC[a],*,
Chanele Polenz, BSc Candidate[b]

KEYWORDS

- Colorectal cancer • Adjuvant chemotherapy • Time to treatment • Wait times
- Treatment barriers

KEY POINTS

- Surgery and adjuvant chemotherapy is the standard of care for all high-risk stage II and all stage II patients with colorectal cancer.
- Research clearly indicates that the timing to the initiation of adjuvant chemotherapy is critical.
- Both clinical and systemic barriers to timely treatment exist: most notably postsurgical complications and care pathway wait times.

BACKGROUND

Colorectal cancer (CRC) is one of the most commonly diagnosed cancers globally in both men and women. Based on the most recent global cancer statistics, an estimated 1.2 million new CRC cases were diagnosed in 2008, with 608,700 patients dying of the disease.[1] The highest incidence rates are found in the developed world, where risk factors such as obesity, poor dietary choices, and physical inactivity are most prevalent.[1–3] In Canada, an estimated 23,300 new CRC cases and 9,200 deaths are estimated to have occurred in 2012.[4] CRC has consequently been the focus for many new screening and treatment initiatives to improve patient care.

Optimizing CRC care is imperative for improving overall survival (OS) and disease-free survival (DFS) rates. As with many solid tumors, the cornerstone of curative CRC treatment is surgical resection. Surgical techniques for resection vary depending on the tumor location and characteristics; however, it is recommended that all colorectal tumors are removed en bloc.[5] Because colorectal tumors often extend into

Disclosures: There are no disclosures to report.
[a] St Michael's Hospital, 30 Bond Street, Room 2081, Toronto, Ontario M5B 1W8, Canada;
[b] University of Waterloo, Ontario, Canada
* Corresponding author.
E-mail address: brezdenc@smh.ca

neighboring structures, en bloc removal maximizes the curative potential of surgery, as well as aiding in the staging process.[5]

In addition to optimal surgery, governing cancer institutions' guidelines also state that patients with high-risk stage II and all patients with stage III CRC are candidates for adjuvant chemotherapy (AC) treatment.[6–9] This article explores the types of chemotherapy available for patients with CRC, the critical issue of timing of AC, and the barriers to treatment.

AC FOR COLORECTAL CANCER

Although surgery is the mainstay of CRC treatment, AC is also an important aspect of increasing DFS and OS. The role of AC is to eradicate micrometastatic tumor deposits, which can increase the chance of cancer recurrence. Recommendations regarding the role and type of AC for patients with CRC have evolved greatly in the past 20 years because of the growing number of clinical trials searching for more effective treatment.

One of the first chemotherapy regimens that showed a definitive DFS benefit in patients with CRC was 5-fluorouracil with levamisole.[10] A randomized controlled trial showed that patients with stage III colon cancer who received levamisole with 5-fluorouracil had a significant reduction (41%) in the relative risk of cancer recurrence compared with patients who did not receive any chemotherapy.[10] A later study showed similar results for patients with stage II and stage III colon cancer, but failed to show any positive effect for patients with rectal cancer.[11] This chemotherapy regimen remained the standard of care in the 1990s, until 5-fluorouracil and folinic acid (leucovorin) were found to be more beneficial.[12–14] The subsequent QUASAR (Quick and Simple and Reliable) trial determined that patients with stage II CRC also received benefits, although small, from adjuvant treatment with 5-fluorouracil and folinic acid.[15] As a result, this established the basis for offering AC to high-risk patients with stage II CRC.

In 2004, the MOSAIC (Multicenter International Study of Oxaliplatin/5-Fluorouracil/Leucovorin [FOLFOX] in the Adjuvant Treatment of Colon Cancer) study further enhanced the treatment regimen, showing that the addition of oxaliplatin to 5-fluorouracil plus leucovorin improved DFS.[16] Although the FOLFOX regimen in the MOSAIC study has proven efficacy, administration of this chemotherapy is not ideal: each cycle is composed of a 2-hour infusion of leucovorin and oxaliplatin, followed by a bolus of 5-fluorouracil, and then a 22-hour infusion of 5-fluorouracil on 2 consecutive days every 2 weeks, for a total of 12 cycles.[16] Furthermore, the X-ACT trial found oral capecitabine (Xeloda) to be an equally effective chemotherapeutic option to 5-fluorouracil and leucovorin, although still less effective than FOLFOX.[17] Hence, common AC for high-risk patients with stage II and all stage III CRC is either FOLFOX or capecitabine, unless drug reactions or comorbidities dictate otherwise.

Chemotherapy regimens vary slightly in patients with rectal cancers compared with patients with colon cancers. Patients with rectal cancer also receive neoadjuvant chemotherapy combined with radiation therapy, because this has been found to increase local control of the tumor (thereby increasing the rate of curative surgery) and increase the number of sphincter preservations in patients with low-lying tumors.[18] However, chemotherapy is commonly continued after surgery, and treatment types are like those available for patients with colon cancer.

In recent years, targeted molecular therapies have also gained prominence as cancer treatment options in combination with chemotherapy. One such drug, bevacizumab (Avastin), is a monoclonal antibody against vascular endothelial growth factor (VEGF), and thus is an antiangiogenic agent that helps suppress tumor growth.[19,20] This targeted therapy yields the greatest benefit when used in combination with chemotherapy in patients with metastatic CRC.[19,20] Another antiangiogenic agent, aflibercept (Zaltrap), has been approved for use in metastatic CRC,[21] but many oral VEGF inhibitor therapies have yet to show any improvement in progression-free survival.[22,23] Anti–epidermal growth factor receptor therapy has also been explored, with cetuximab and panitumumab showing promise for patients with metastatic CRC who have the wild-type KRAS gene.[24–26] However, to date these targeted therapies have not shown benefit in the adjuvant setting.[27–29] Current clinical trials are underway to investigate optimal sequencing strategies in combination with chemotherapy as novel molecular targeted therapies emerge as the forerunners in the future of cancer treatments.

TIMING OF AC: IS IT IMPORTANT?

Based on the aforementioned studies, current governing health institutions recommend that all high-risk stage II and all stage III patients with CRC receive AC, ideally within 8 weeks of surgical resection.[6–9] In Canada, government health agencies responsible for improving provincial cancer care, such as Cancer Care Ontario (CCO), mandate treatment timelines. In addition to the overall 8-week treatment timeline, CCO advises that Ontario cancer centers should aim for the following wait times: time from surgeon's referral to medical oncology consult should be no longer than 14 days, and medical oncology consult to the start of AC treatment should be no longer than 28 days.[30] However, these timelines are arbitrary, set on the basis that most clinical trials randomize patients to a treatment arm and begin AC within 6 to 8 weeks after surgical resection.

Animal and mathematical modeling, in addition to human molecular-based studies, have provided strong clues that the timing of AC is important. Research in animals has shown that the surgical removal of tumors may stimulate an increase in the number of residual tumor cells by prompting the conversion of arrested (G0) cells into a cycling phase.[31] There is similar evidence that the surgical resection of tumors may activate dormant distant metastasis and the stimulation of angiogenesis via the release of circulating factors.[32,33] Research also suggests that major surgery can trigger altered host defense mechanisms, in which cytotoxic T cells and natural killer cell activity are suppressed, facilitating the proliferation of micrometastatic sites.[34,35] These data suggest that the time between surgery and the start of AC is critical in preventing the development of metastatic cancer. Mathematical modeling based on empirical data has indicated the same concept: that the probability of eradicating micrometastatic cancer after surgical resection is inversely proportional to the tumor burden that remains to be destroyed, and consequently is inversely proportional to the time from surgery to AC.[36] Based on this model, the window of opportunity to eradicate these metastatic sites is 100 days, after which the curative potential of AC has been surpassed.[36]

The issue of optimal timing between surgery and AC has also been studied for other tumor sites. Studies have shown that patients with breast cancer who start AC beyond 4 months (12 weeks) after surgery show a marked decrease in the effectiveness of their therapy.[37,38] The International Breast Cancer Study Group also investigated the matter of optimal timing of AC; their research suggested that ER-negative, premenopausal patients experienced a significant increase in DFS when AC commenced within 20 days of surgery compared with patients who commenced AC within 21 to 86 days of surgery.[39] A more encompassing meta-analysis of patients with breast cancer also found that a 4-week delay in time to AC was significantly associated with a decrease in OS and DFS.[40] These studies, although focused on another tumor type, also provide strong evidence that the timing of AC is essential in achieving optimal DFS.

The association between the timing of AC and CRC outcomes has also been increasingly studied. Several retrospective reviews and prospective trials have corroborated the theory that a delay in the commencement of AC is associated with worse outcomes in patients with CRC; specifically, most studies showed that a delay of greater than 8 to 12 weeks greatly reduces the efficacy of adjuvant treatment.[41–47] However, optimal treatment times were not well studied until recently. In a recent meta-analysis, Biagi and colleagues[48] investigated the correlation between time to AC and survival outcomes in patients with CRC; an analysis of 10 studies (7 published articles, 3 abstracts) involving 15,410 patients yielded an association between longer wait times to AC and worse survival outcomes. Their findings also suggest that relative OS decreases by 14% for every 4-week delay to the initiation of treatment.[48] Based on these results, AC treatment should optimally begin within 4 to 6 weeks of surgical resection.

Timely AC treatment is imperative in improving patient outcomes. As such, some hospitals have begun to investigate their institutional wait times for AC following surgical resection. A recent retrospective review conducted as St Michael's Hospital (SMH), an inner-city academic Toronto hospital, sought to investigate hospital wait times and elucidate barriers to timely AC treatment.[49] Only 37.1% of patients at SMH were treated within the timeline of 4 to 6 weeks recommended by Biagi and colleagues,[48,49] and the wait time between surgery and first AC treatment averaged 50.4 days (7.2 weeks).[49] A larger retrospective study, which included patients from both SMH and Mount Sinai Hospital in Toronto, found similar results: the mean time from surgery to first AC treatment was 8.2 weeks.[50] Based on these results, steps need to be taken to reduce the time between surgical resection and AC in order to improve outcomes for patients with CRC.

CHALLENGES AND BARRIERS TO AC

There are several barriers that may delay the start of adjuvant treatment. There are both clinical and systemic challenges to initiating therapy. Among clinical barriers to treatment, age and socioeconomic factors seem to present the biggest challenges to timely treatment.[42,51,52] As with any treatment decision, patient preference may also play a role in the time to initiation of AC.

However, perhaps one of the biggest challenges to timely AC treatment is the presence of postoperative complications, which prolong patient recovery times. Several studies have shown that surgical complications, such as problems with wound healing, are significantly associated with delays to the initiation of AC.[42,49–53] Furthermore, surgical complications have also been linked to worse OS and DFS.[53] As a result, efforts have been made to encourage surgical research designed to minimize these complications and optimize patient care during recovery. For example, a recent study found that the use of a Pfannenstiel incision, commonly used in gynecologic surgery, is associated with a minimized risk of postsurgical would complications in minimally invasive CRC surgery.[54]

Efforts should also be made to properly counsel patients regarding modifiable factors that could affect their surgical outcomes. For example, proper nutrition before surgery and early initiation of enteral feeding after surgery have both been shown to minimize hospital stay and shorten recovery times after surgical resection.[55–59] Smoking and alcohol cessation have also been attributed to better surgical outcomes.[60] It is also important that diabetic patients are well controlled, because poor postoperative glycemic control has been associated with an increase in surgical site infections.[61] Thus, it is critical that postoperative recovery pathways are in place to minimize surgical healing times, and hence allow patients to begin AC as soon as possible.

Systemic barriers, primarily institutional wait times, also play a key role in delaying the start of AC. A retrospective review conducted at an inner-city Toronto hospital identified the time from surgery to medical oncology referral, time awaiting port-a-cath or central venous access device insertion for the AC treatment infusion, and time from medical oncology consult to first AC as significant systemic barriers to timely treatment.[49] These wait times may also depend on other factors, such as the time to procure a pathology report, which could be optimized by critically evaluating the clinical care pathway. For example, institutions with on-site pathology laboratories may receive pathology results more quickly than those who depend on outside laboratories. These significant wait times also clearly indicated the importance of timely referrals among health care professionals, and also highlight the need for a cohesive, multidisciplinary, team-based approach to oncology care. The introduction of multidisciplinary cancer conferences (MCCs) has improved the communication between cancer-treating physicians, engaging all health care professionals involved in the patient's cancer care pathway. These MCCs are usually weekly meetings of surgeons, medical oncologists, radiation oncologists, pathologists, and radiologists who discuss cancer cases to ensure that optimal treatment is recommended based on current treatment guidelines.

Delays in initiation of treatment may also be related to physician or patient indecision and reluctance. Maintaining dose-intense regimens is efficacious, and dose modifications may detract from the full benefits of chemotherapy.[62–67] As such, physicians may delay the start of treatment until they are confident that patients are well enough to begin a treatment at full dose intensity, to increase the chances of receiving the full benefits of AC.

Physicians may also be reluctant to administer chemotherapy to elderly patients, because patients more than 70 years old are often underrepresented in clinical trials (most CRC trials have an age exclusion of greater than 71–75 years),[12,16,17,68] and thus the results may be difficult to extrapolate to the older patient population. This underrepresentation is surprising, because the median age of patients with CRC is 63 to 65 years; this disease is a disease of the elderly. However, age should not be seen as a barrier to treatment; physiologic age, rather than biological age, is a better predictor of treatment tolerance. The functional status of elderly patients more than 70 years of age should be assessed in collaboration with geriatric oncologists when discussing chemotherapy treatment, preferably by the use of a comprehensive geriatric assessment.[69–71] For this reason, it is up to the physician's discretion as to how best to administer the chemotherapy for their patients' greatest benefit.

Some studies have begun to explore the issue of chemotherapy regimens for elderly patients. A prospective study of 844 patients with CRC found that patients older than 70 years in good performance status tolerated 5-fluorouracil-containing therapies just as well as younger patients, with similar beneficial outcomes.[72] A recent phase III trial, AVEX, also evaluated the safety and efficacy of capecitabine with bevacizumab for patients with metastatic CRC more than 70 years of age, and showed that this chemotherapy regimen was well tolerated and safe with improvements in survival.[73] Finally, a patient's indecision to begin a chemotherapy regimen may also factor into the delay to AC.

SUMMARY

AC has shown to improve the risk of recurrence and mortality of CRC, but there have been no advances in adjuvant CRC chemotherapy since FOLFOX in 2004. Furthermore, although novel molecular targeted therapies have recently been developed, none have yet shown any evidence of benefit in the adjuvant setting. Timely adminis-tration of AC plays a critical role in improving OS and DFS in patients with CRC. Cur-rent evidence strongly suggests that delays in treatment, especially beyond 4 to 8 weeks from surgery, negatively affect outcomes. Several clinical and systemic bar-riers to treatment have been identified, and efforts should be made to overcome institution-specific challenges to timely AC. Further research is warranted on care pathways and other potential strategies for overcoming barriers to timely treatment.

REFERENCES

1. Jemal A, Bray F, Center MM, et al. Global cancer statistics. CA Cancer J Clin 2011;61:69–90.
2. Boyle P, Levin B, editors. World cancer report 2008. Lyon (France): World Health Organization, International Agency for Research on Cancer; 2008.
3. Ferrari P, Jenab M, Norat T, et al. Lifetime and baseline alcohol intake and risk of colon and rectal cancers in the European prospective investigation into cancer and nutrition (EPIC). Int J Cancer 2007;121:2065–72.
4. Canadian Cancer Society's Steering Committee on Cancer Statistics. Canadian cancer statistics 2012. Toronto: Canadian Cancer Society; 2012.
5. Nelson H, Petrelli N, Carlin A, et al. Guidelines 2000 for colon and rectal cancer surgery. J Natl Cancer Inst 2001;93:583–96.
6. National Institutes of Health. Adjuvant therapy for patients with colon and rectum cancer: NIH consensus statement, vol. 8. Bethesda (MD): National Institutes of Health; 1990. p. 1–25.
7. Benson AB III, Schrag D, Somerfield MR, et al. American Society of Clinical Oncology recommendations on adjuvant chemotherapy for stage II colon cancer. J Clin Oncol 2004;22:3408–19.
8. Figueredo A, Charette ML, Maroun J, et al. Adjuvant therapy for stage II colon cancer: a systematic review from the Cancer Care Ontario Program in Evidence-based Care's Gastrointestinal Cancer Disease Site Group. J Clin Oncol 2004;22:3395–407.
9. Jonker D, Spithoff K, Maroun J. Adjuvant systemic chemotherapy for stage II and III colon cancer following complete surgical resection. Program in Evidence-based Care (PEBC), Cancer Care Ontario (CCO). Conducted April 17, 2008. Evidence-based series 2–29. In review.
10. Moertel CG, Fleming TR, Macdonald JS, et al. Levamisole and fluorouracil for adjuvant therapy of resected colon carcinoma. N Engl J Med 1990;322:352–8.
11. Taal BG, van Tinteren H, Zoetmulder FA, et al. Adjuvant 5FU plus levamisole in colonic or rectal cancer: improved survival in stage II and III. Br J Cancer 2001; 85:1437–43.
12. Wolmark N, Rockette H, Mamounas E, et al. Clinical trial to assess the relative efficacy of fluorouracil and leucovorin, fluorouracil and levamisole and fluoro-uracil, leucovorin, and levamisole in patients with Dukes B and C carcinoma of the colon: results from National Surgical Adjuvant Breast and Bowel Project C-04. J Clin Oncol 1999;17:3553–9.
13. O'Connell MJ, Laurie JA, Kahn M, et al. Prospectively randomized trial of post-operative adjuvant chemotherapy in patients with high-risk colon cancer. J Clin Oncol 1998;16:295–300.
14. Haller DG, Catalano PJ, MacDonald JS, et al. Phase III study of fluorouracil, leu-covorin, and levamisole (LEV) in high-risk stage II and III colon cancer: final report of Intergroup 0089. J Clin Oncol 2005;23:8671–8.

15. Quasar Collaborative Group. Adjuvant chemotherapy versus observation in patients with colorectal cancer: a randomized study. Lancet 2007;370:2020–9.
16. Andre T, Boni C, Mounedji-Boudiaf L, et al. Oxaliplatin, fluorouracil, and leucovorin as adjuvant treatment for colon cancer. N Engl J Med 2004;350:2343–51.
17. Twelves C, Scheithauer W, McKendrick J, et al. Capecitabine versus 5-fluorouracil/folinic acid as adjuvant therapy for stage III colon cancer: final results from the X-ACT trial with analysis by age and preliminary evidence of a pharmacodynamic marker of efficacy. Ann Oncol 2011. http://dx.doi.org/10.1093/annonc/mdr366.
18. Sauer R, Becker H, Hohenberger W, et al. Preoperative versus postoperative chemoradiotherapy for rectal cancer. N Engl J Med 2004;351:1731–40.
19. Hurwitz H, Fehrenbacher L, Novotny W, et al. Bevacizumab plus irinotecan, fluorouracil, and leucovorin for metastatic colorectal cancer. N Engl J Med 2004; 350:2335–42.
20. Saltz LB, Clarke S, Diaz-Rubio E, et al. Bevacizumab in combination with oxaliplatin-based chemotherapy as first-line therapy in metastatic colorectal cancer: a randomized phase III study. J Clin Oncol 2008;26:2013–9.
21. Van Cutsem E, Tabernero J, Lakomy R, et al. Addition of aflibercept to fluorouracil, leucovorin, and irinotecan improves survival in a phase III randomized trial in patients with metastatic colorectal cancer previously treated with an oxaliplatin-based regimen. J Clin Oncol 2012;30:3499–506.
22. Hecht JR, Trarbach T, Jaeger E, et al. A randomized, double-blind, placebo-controlled, phase III study in patients (Pts) with metastatic adenocarcinoma of the colon or rectum receiving first-line chemotherapy with oxaliplatin/5-fluorouracil/leucovorin and PTK787/ZK 222584 or placebo (CONFIRM-1) 2005 ASCO Annual Meeting Proceedings. J Clin Oncol 2005;23:16S [abstract LBA3].
23. Saltz LB, Rosen LS, Marshall JL, et al. Phase II trial of sunitinib in patients with metastatic colorectal cancer after failure of standard therapy. J Clin Oncol 2007; 25:4793–9.
24. Saltz LB, Meropol NJ, Loehrer PJ Sr, et al. Phase II trial of cetuximab in patients with refractory colorectal cancer that expresses the epidermal growth factor receptor. J Clin Oncol 2004;22:1201–8.
25. Lievre A, Bachet JB, Boige V, et al. KRAS mutations as an independent prognostic factor in patients with advanced colorectal cancer treated with cetuximab. J Clin Oncol 2008;26:374–9.
26. Gibson TB, Ranganathan A, Grothey A. Randomized phase III trial results of panitumumab, a fully human anti-epidermal growth factor receptor monoclonal antibody, in metastatic colorectal cancer. Clin Colorectal Cancer 2006;6:29–31.
27. de Gramont A, Van Cutsem E, Schmoll HJ, et al. Bevacizumab plus oxaliplatin-based chemotherapy as adjuvant treatment for colon cancer (AVANT): a phase 3 randomised controlled trial. Lancet Oncol 2012;13:1225–33.
28. Allegra CJ, Yothers G, O'Connell MJ, et al. Bevacizumab in stage II-III colon cancer: 5-year update of the National Surgical Adjuvant Breast and Bowel Project C-08 trial. J Clin Oncol 2013;31:359–64.
29. Alberts SR, Sargent DJ, Nair S, et al. Effect of oxaliplatin, fluorouracil, and leucovorin with or without cetuximab on survival among patients with resected stage III colon cancer: a randomized trial. JAMA 2012;307:1381–93.
30. Systemic treatment wait times. Cancer Care Ontario, Action Cancer Ontario. Available at: http://www.cancercare.on.ca/cms/One.aspx?portalId=1377&pageId=8888. Accessed April 19, 2013.

31. Gunduz N, Fisher B, Saffer EA. Effect of surgical removal on the growth and kinetics of residual tumor. Cancer Res 1979;39:3861–5.

32. Baum M, Demicheli R, Hrushesky W, et al. Does surgery unfavourably perturb the "natural history" of early breast cancer by accelerating the appearance of distant metastases? Eur J Cancer 2005;41:508–15.

33. Fisher B, Gunduz N, Coyle J, et al. Presence of a growth-stimulating factor in serum following primary tumor removal in mice. Cancer Res 1989;49: 1996–2001.

34. Hensler T, Hecker H, Heeg K, et al. Distinct mechanisms of immunosuppression as a consequence of major surgery. Infect Immun 1997;65:2283–91.

35. Stalder M, Birsan T, Hausen B, et al. Immunosuppressive effects of surgery assessed by flow cytometry in nonhuman primates after nephrectomy. Transpl Int 2005;18:1158–65.

36. Harless W, Qiu Y. Cancer: a medical emergency. Med Hypotheses 2006;67: 1054–9.

37. Lohrisch C, Paltiel C, Gelmon K, et al. Impact on survival of time from definitive surgery to initiation of adjuvant chemotherapy for early-stage breast cancer. J Clin Oncol 2006;24:4888–94.

38. Hershman DL, Wang X, McBride R, et al. Delay of adjuvant chemotherapy initiation following breast cancer surgery among elderly women. Breast Cancer Res Treat 2006;99:313–21.

39. Colleoni M, Bonetti M, Coates AS, et al. Early start of adjuvant chemotherapy may improve treatment outcome for premenopausal breast cancer patients with tumors not expressing estrogen receptors. The International Breast Cancer Study Group. J Clin Oncol 2000;18:584–90.

40. Yu KD, Huang S, Zhang JX, et al. Association between delayed initiation of adjuvant CMF or anthracycline-based chemotherapy and survival in breast cancer: a systematic review and meta-analysis. BMC Cancer 2013. http://dx.doi.org/10. 1186/1471-2407-13-240.

41. Ahmed S, Ahmad I, Zhu T, et al. Early discontinuation but not the timing of adjuvant therapy affects survival of patients with high-risk colorectal cancer: a population-based study. Dis Colon Rectum 2010;53:1432–8.

42. Cheung WY, Neville BA, Earle CC. Etiology of delays in the initiation of adjuvant chemotherapy and their impact on outcomes for stage II and III rectal cancer. Dis Colon Rectum 2009;52:1054–63.

43. Hershman D, Hall MJ, Wang X, et al. Timing of adjuvant chemotherapy initiation after surgery for stage III colon cancer. Cancer 2006;107:2581–8.

44. Czaykowski PM, Gill S, Kennecke HF, et al. Adjuvant chemotherapy for stage III colon cancer: does timing matter? Dis Colon Rectum 2011;54:1082–9.

45. Lima IS, Yasui Y, Scarfe A, et al. Association between receipt and timing of adjuvant chemotherapy and survival for patients with stage III colon cancer in Alberta, Canada. Cancer 2011;117:3833–40.

46. Bayraktar UD, Chen E, Bayraktar S, et al. Does delay of adjuvant chemotherapy impact survival in patients with resected stage II and III colon adenocarcinoma? Cancer 2011;117:2364–70.

47. Berglund A, Cedermark B, Glimelius B. Is it deleterious to delay the start of adjuvant chemotherapy in colon cancer stage III? Ann Oncol 2008;19: 400–2.

48. Biagi JJ, Raphael MJ, Mackillop WJ, et al. Association between time to initiation of adjuvant chemotherapy and survival in colorectal cancer: a systematic review and meta-analysis. JAMA 2011;305:2335–42.

49. Marchand C, Ebrahim J, Hassan M, et al. Time from surgery to first adjuvant chemotherapy: experiences at an inner-city Canadian hospital. J Clin Oncol 2012;30(Suppl 34). [Abstract 527].

50. Polenz C, Manoharan A, Sevick L, et al. Time from surgery to first adjuvant chemotherapy: experiences at two Toronto hospitals. J Clin Oncol 2013; 31(Suppl) [abstract e17557].

51. Hendren S, Birkmeyer JD, Yin H, et al. Surgical complications are associated with omission of chemotherapy for stage III colorectal cancer. Dis Colon Rectum 2010;53:1587–93.

52. Van der Geest LG, Portielje JE, Wouters MW, et al. Complicated postoperative recovery increases omission, delay and discontinuation of adjuvant chemotherapy in patients with colon cancer stage III. Colorectal Dis 2013. http://dx.doi.org/10.1111/codi.12288.

53. Law WL, Choi HK, Lee YM, et al. The impact of postoperative complications on long-term outcomes following curative resection for colorectal cancer. Ann Surg Oncol 2007;14:2559–66.

54. Orcutt ST, Balentine CJ, Marshall TL, et al. Use of a Pfannenstiel incision in minimally invasive colorectal cancer surgery is associated with a lower risk of wound complications. Tech Coloproctol 2012;16:127–32.

55. Hill GL. Changes in body composition and outcome in surgical patients. Clin Nutr 1994;13:331–40.

56. Kehlet H, Wilmore DW. Multimodal strategies to improve surgical outcome. Am J Surg 2002;183:630–44.

57. Lewis SJ, Egger M, Sylvester PA, et al. Early enteral feeding versus "nil by mouth" after gastrointestinal surgery: systematic review and meta-analysis of controlled trials. BMJ 2001;323:773–6.

58. Henriksen MG, Hansen HV, Hessov I. Early oral nutrition after elective colorectal surgery: influence of balanced analgesia and enforced mobilization. Nutrition 2002;18:263–7.

59. Fearon KC, Luff R. The nutritional management of surgical patients: enhanced recovery after surgery. Proc Nutr Soc 2003;62:807–11.

60. Sorenson LT, Jorgensen T, Kirkeby LT, et al. Smoking and alcohol abuse are major risk factors for anastomotic leakage in colorectal surgery. Br J Surg 1999;86:927–31.

61. McConnell YJ, Johnson PM, Porter GA. Surgical site infections following colorectal surgery in patients with diabetes: association with postoperative hyperglycemia. J Gastrointest Surg 2009;13:508–15.

62. Buroker TR, O'Connell MJ, Wieand S, et al. Randomized comparison of two schedules of fluorouracil and leucovorin in the treatment of advanced colorectal cancer. J Clin Oncol 1994;12:14–20.

63. De Gramont A, Bosset JF, Milan C, et al. Randomized trial comparing monthly low-dose leucovorin and fluorouracil bolus with bimonthly continuous infusion for advanced colorectal cancer: a French Intergroup study. J Clin Oncol 1997;15:808–15.

64. Weh HJ, Zschaber R, Braumann D, et al. A randomised phase III study comparing weekly folinic acid (FA) and high dose 5-fluorouracil (5-FU) with monthly 5-FU/FA d 1-5 in untreated patients with metastatic colorectal carcinoma (CRC). Ann Oncol 1998;9:33.

65. Kerr DJ, Gray R, McConkey C, et al. Adjuvant chemotherapy with 5-fluorouracil, L-folinic acid and levamisole for patients with colorectal cancer: non-randomised comparison of weekly versus four-weekly schedules – less pain, same gain. Ann Oncol 2000;11:947–55.

66. Wood WC, Budman DR, Korzun AH, et al. Dose and dose intensity of adjuvant chemotherapy for stage II, node-positive breast carcinoma. N Engl J Med 1994; 330:1253–9.

67. Bonadonna G, Valagussa P, Moliterni A, et al. Adjuvant cyclophosphamide, methotrexate, and fluorouracil in node-positive breast cancer. N Engl J Med 1995;332:901–6.

68. Hutchins LF, Unger JM, Crowley JJ, et al. Underrepresentation of patients 65 years of age or older in cancer-treatment trials. N Engl J Med 1999;341:2061–7.

69. Caillet P, Canoui-Poitrine F, Vouriot J, et al. Comprehensive geriatric assessment in the decision-making process in elderly patients with cancer: ELCAPA study. J Clin Oncol 2011;29:3636–42.

70. Hamaker ME, Jonker JM, de Rooij SE, et al. Frailty screening methods for predicting outcome of a comprehensive geriatric assessment in elderly patients with cancer: a systematic review. Lancet Oncol 2012;13:e437–44. http://dx.doi.org/10.1016/S1470-2045(12)70259-0.

71. Aaldriks AA, Maartense E, le Cessie S, et al. Predictive value of geriatric assessment for patients older than 70 years, treated with chemotherapy. Crit Rev Oncol Hematol 2011;79:205–12.

72. Popescu RA, Norman A, Ross PJ, et al. Adjuvant or palliative chemotherapy for colorectal cancer in patients 70 years or older. J Clin Oncol 1999;17:2412–8.

73. Cunningham D, Lang I, Lorusso V, et al. Bevacizumab (bev) in combination with capecitabine (cape) for the first-line treatment of elderly patients with metastatic colorectal cancer (mCRC): results of a randomized international phase III trial (AVEX). J Clin Oncol 2012;30(Suppl 34) [abstract 337].

Imaging in Rectal Cancer
Magnetic Resonance Imaging Versus Endorectal Ultrasonography

Tushar Samdani, MD[a], Julio Garcia-Aguilar, MD, PhD[b],*

KEYWORDS

- Rectal cancer • Endorectal ultrasonography • Magnetic resonance imaging
- Circumferential resection margin • Tumor staging

KEY POINTS

- Endorectal ultrasonography (ERUS) provides excellent visualization of the layers of the bowel wall; magnetic resonance imaging (MRI) does not.
- ERUS provides better visualization of superficial tumors; MRI provides better visualization of locally advanced or stenotic tumors.
- MRI and ERUS are complementary tools in evaluation of lymph nodes.
- MRI is best at visualizing the circumferential resection margin.

INTRODUCTION

In the last decades, we have seen dramatic improvements in the outcomes of patients with rectal cancer. The rate of local recurrence has decreased, the probability of survival has increased, and the quality of life has improved. Advances in surgical pathology, which have added to our understanding of the causes of locoregional recurrences, refinements in surgical techniques, and the widespread use of neoadjuvant therapy, have all contributed to these improvements. However, advances in imaging have also played a pivotal role in identifying those at risk for recurrence, helping in planning surgical procedures and selecting patients for neoadjuvant therapy. Adequate imaging is a fundamental component of rectal cancer management.

Preoperative evaluation of the patient with rectal cancer goes beyond determination of tumor stage. Treatment planning requires not only defining the depth of tumor invasion in relation to the bowel wall, and the presence of metastatic regional lymph nodes, but also the precise relationship of tumor to other pelvic structures such as

[a] Memorial Sloan-Kettering Cancer Center, 1275 York Avenue, New York, NY 10065, USA;
[b] Colorectal Service, Department of Surgery, Memorial Sloan-Kettering Cancer Center, 1275 York Avenue, Room C-1067, New York, NY 10065, USA
* Corresponding author.
E-mail address: garciaaj@mskcc.org

Surg Oncol Clin N Am 23 (2014) 59–77
http://dx.doi.org/10.1016/j.soc.2013.09.011
1055-3207/14/$ – see front matter © 2014 Elsevier Inc. All rights reserved.

the mesorectal fascia, the levator muscle, the anal sphincters, and adjacent organs. In addition, assessment of the pelvic nodal basins outside the mesorectal fascia, and assessment of the retroperitoneal nodes, liver, and lungs, can provide useful information that may affect the treatment strategy.

Magnetic resonance imaging (MRI), endorectal ultrasonography (ERUS), and computed tomography (CT) are the imaging modalities most commonly used in evaluation of the patient with rectal cancer. Each has unique strengths and limitations. Rather than being used in the locoregional staging of rectal cancer, CT scanning is mainly used to exclude distant metastasis, and will not be reviewed here.

MRI of the rectum can be performed with either an endorectal coil or a phased-array surface coil. Endorectal coil MRI yields high-resolution images of the layers of the rectal wall, although clear differentiation between the mucosa and submucosa remains difficult. However, endorectal coil MRI provides only limited views of the rectum, cannot be used in the setting of stenotic or high tumors, and is poorly tolerated by patients. Therefore, endorectal coil MRI is not commonly used in the evaluation of rectal cancer and is not discussed in this review. Rectal MRI with a phased-array surface coil does not depict the layers of the bowel wall; however, it yields large field, high-resolution images of the rectum and other pelvic structures and is now an essential tool in the preoperative evaluation of rectal cancer. ERUS is a simple, widely available office procedure that provides high-resolution images of the rectal wall and surrounding tissues, within a short focal range. Because ERUS depicts the different layers of the bowel wall, it is useful in staging early rectal cancer; however, given its short focal range, it is not accurate in assessing the relationship of more advanced tumors to important anatomic structures, such as the mesorectal fascia. Thus, MRI, ERUS, and CT should be seen as complementary rather than competing tools, each providing unique and important information in the evaluation of the patient with rectal cancer.

In this article, an overview is provided of the anatomy of the rectum and other pelvic structures relevant to the preoperative evaluation and surgical treatment of rectal cancer. We then review the technical aspects, applications, and limitations of MRI and ERUS, the imaging modalities commonly used in preoperative assessment.

RELEVANT ANATOMY

The rectum corresponds to the distal portion of the large bowel, but neither its beginning nor end is sharply defined by specific anatomic landmarks. Proximally, the sigmoid colon transitions into the rectum at the rectosigmoid junction, located approximately 12 to 15 cm from the anal verge. The relationship of the large bowel with the promontory, often considered the beginning of the rectum, is variable, because it depends on the laxity of the mesorectum. Distally, the rectum transitions into the anal canal at the level of the anorectal ring, a palpable anatomic landmark corresponding to the impromptu of the puborectalis on the bowel wall. The anal canal extends from the anorectal ring to the anal verge, the palpable groove between the distal edge of the internal sphincter and the subcutaneous portion of the external sphincter. The location of a rectal tumor is best determined by measuring the distance of the lower edge of tumor from the anal verge, using a rigid proctoscope. This permits simultaneous viewing of the tumor, the anal verge, and the measuring marks on the instrument. However, measurements obtained from high quality sagittal images can also provide a good estimate of the distance of the tumor from the anal verge.

Similar to other segments of the gastrointestinal tract, the rectal wall is composed of a mucosa, a, submucosa, and a muscularis layer. The muscularis propria of the rectum has an inner circular layer, which, close to the anus, becomes the internal sphincter, and an outer longitudinal layer, which, at the level of the anal canal, forms the conjoined longitudinal muscle between the internal and external sphincter. In the anterior aspect of the upper and mid rectum, the muscularis is covered by peritoneum. In the remainder of the rectum, the muscularis is in contact with the perirectal-mesorectal fat. The different layers of the bowel wall are best visualized on ERUS (**Fig. 1**).

The upper portion of the rectum is located above the anterior peritoneal reflection and is covered with peritoneum in the front and on both sides. Posteriorly, the upper rectum is attached to the concavity of the sacrum by a mesentery, the mesorectum, which is a continuation of the mesentery of the sigmoid colon. Below the peritoneal reflection, the rectum is completely extraperitoneal and fully surrounded by mesorectum.

The mesorectum, the visceral mesentery of the rectum derived from the dorsal mesentery of the hindgut, contains the terminal branches of the superior rectal vessels and the lymphatic drainage of the rectum. The mesorectum is covered by a thin, glistening membrane called the mesorectal fascia. The mesorectum extends posteriorly from the promontory to Waldeyer's fascia, a condensation of connective tissue spanning the area from the fourth sacral vertebra to the anorectal ring (**Fig. 2**). Posteriorly, the mesorectum is separated from the presacral fascia by an avascular plane of loose areolar tissue. The plane between the mesorectal fascia and the presacral fascia is the natural plane of dissection during a total mesorectal excision (TME).

The mesorectum is thick posteriorly, where it has a characteristic bilobular appearance. However, anteriorly, it is either absent (in the upper intraperitoneal portion of the rectum) or reduced to a thin layer of areolar tissue (in the mid and distal rectum). The mesorectal fascia is not as well defined anteriorly as it is posteriorly (**Fig. 3**). In the front, the thin mesorectum is separated from the urogenital organs by a remnant of the fusion of 2 layers of the embryologic peritoneal cul-de-sac known as Denonvillier's fascia, which is not well visualized in imaging studies. MRI provides excellent visualization of the seminal vesicles and prostate. The relationship of the rectal wall with seminal vesicles, prostate, and vagina is also well visualized on ERUS (**Fig. 4**).

The mesorectum tapers off distally as the rectum funnels down toward the anorectal ring, where the longitudinal layer of the muscularis propria of the rectum is in direct contact with the levator muscle. The proximity of the rectal wall to the levator muscle

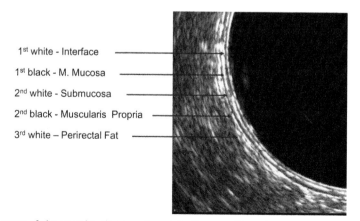

1st white - Interface
1st black - M. Mucosa
2nd white - Submucosa
2nd black - Muscularis Propria
3rd white – Perirectal Fat

Fig. 1. Layers of the rectal wall on endorectal ultrasound imaging.

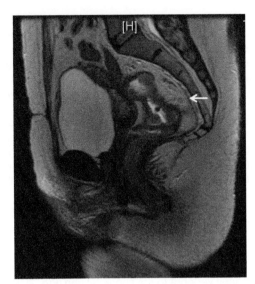

Fig. 2. Sagittal T2-weigted view of the pelvis in a female patient with rectal cancer. The *arrow* points to the posterior aspect of the mesorectal fascia. The areolar space between the mesorectal fascia and the presacral fascia corresponds to the dissection plane followed during the total mesorectal excision.

must be taken into consideration when deciding between an abdominoperineal excision or a sphincter-sparing procedure, in the setting of transmural rectal cancers located at or below the level of the anorectal ring. Below the peritoneal reflection, the mesorectum intermingles on both sides of the pelvis with a condensation of connective tissue surrounding the autonomic nerves that pass from the pelvic plexus to the rectum. These bilateral condensations of the endopelvic fascia are known as

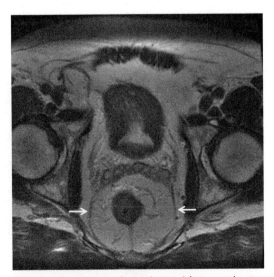

Fig. 3. Axial view of the pelvis in a male patient with an early stage rectal cancer on T2-weighted imaging. The *arrows* point to both sides of the mesorectal fascia.

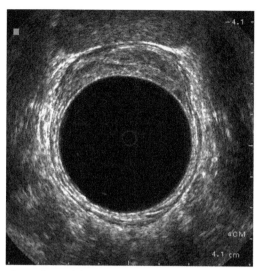

Fig. 4. ERUS image of a patient with an anteriorly located rectal cancer separated from the prostate by a thin hyperechoic rim corresponding to perirectal fat.

lateral ligaments, and connect the pelvic sidewall with the mesorectum. In some individuals, the lateral ligaments contain accessory middle rectal vessels.

The blood supply of the rectum comes primarily from the superior rectal artery, which is the continuation of the inferior mesenteric artery after it gives off the left colic artery. The superior rectal artery gives several sigmoidal branches before diving into the mesorectum, where it gives multiple branches to the rectum. The superior rectal vein has a parallel course to its homonymous artery, on its way to join the left colic vein to form the inferior mesenteric vein draining into the splenic vein. The lower portion of the rectum also receives blood supply from the internal iliac vessels. The middle rectal artery, an inconsistent branch of the inferior vesical artery, is usually located deep in the pelvis, running over the levator muscle toward the distal wall of the rectum. The inferior rectal artery is a branch of the pudendal artery and provides blood supply to the anal canal and anal sphincter. The middle and inferior rectal vessels anastomose with the upper rectal vessels to supply enough blood to the entire rectum. As in other locations, the middle and inferior rectal veins follow the course of the homonymous arteries and drain into systemic circulation through the internal iliac veins. Metastatic lymph nodes in patients with rectal cancer tend to be located in the mesorectum and along the superior rectal vessels, but in some cases, they can be located along the internal iliac vessels. Both MRI and ERUS can show the presence of metastatic lymph nodes, with varying degrees of accuracy (**Fig. 5**).

The autonomic pelvic nerves are rarely visible on imaging studies, but an understanding of their relationship to the anatomical landmarks that are commonly visualized helps in planning the surgical procedure and anticipating postoperative function in patients with locally advanced rectal cancer. The sympathetic plexus is at risk of injury near the origin of the inferior mesenteric artery and at the level of the aortic bifurcation during the dissection and ligation of the superior rectal vessels. The parasympathetic nerves are most at risk during the posterolateral dissection of the mesorectum, close to the lateral ligaments. The neurovascular bundle is most at risk close to the junction of the seminal vesicles, with the lateral aspects of the prostate.

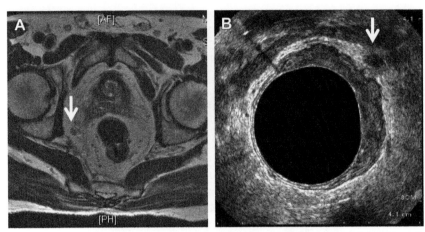

Fig. 5. (*A*) Axial view of the pelvis of a male rectal cancer patient on T2-weighted imaging. The *white arrow* points to an enlarged lymph node – most likely metastatic - in the territory of the internal iliac vessels. The area of intermediate signal intensity in the back of the rectum corresponds to the primary tumor. (*B*) Endorectal ultrasound imaging of a rectal tumor with a mesorectal lymph node. The *white arrow* points to the enlarged lymph node, which is most likely metastatic.

The pelvic floor, also known as the pelvic diaphragm, comprises the levator ani and coccygeus muscles. The levator muscle is a thin, broad layer of muscle that inserts in the inner wall of the pelvis and unites with the muscle of the opposite side to form the greater part of the pelvic diaphragm. The anterior portion inserts in the posterior aspect of the pubic bones lateral to the symphysis, running posteriorly and obliquely to join the perineal body. This muscle is known as the levator prostate (in males) or the pubovaginalis (in females). The next muscular fascicle, known as the puborectalis, extends from the posterior aspect of the pubic bone and loops around the back of the rectum, becoming continuous with the muscle of the opposite side (**Fig. 6**). The lower fibers of the puborectalis intermingle with the fibers of the upper portion of the external sphincter. The ileococcygeus and pubococcygeus insert in the pubis and in the tendinous arch of the obturator fascia, extending obliquely downwards and backwards from/toward the perineal body, the anal sphincter, the anococcygeal ligament, and the coccyx. The levator muscles create a funnel-shaped diaphragm with a central opening delineated by the puborectalis sling and the symphysis of the pubis, which allows passage of the urethra and the rectum in both males and females, and the vagina in females. The coccygeus muscle extends from the spine of the ischium and the sacrospinous ligament and inserts in the coccyx.

TECHNIQUES AND IMAGE INTERPRETATION
MRI

MRI imaging using multiple sequences, with and without contrast, provides excellent anatomical and tissue resolution. The addition of advanced functional MRI sequences such as diffusion-weighted imaging (DWI) and dynamic contrast-enhancement (DCE, or "perfusion") allow for the quantification of tumor biologic processes such as microcirculation, vascular permeability, and tissue cellularity. These images are potentially useful for early assessment of rectal cancer response to neoadjuvant therapy, but are still considered experimental.

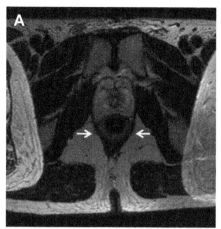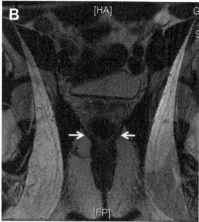

Fig. 6. (*A*) Axial view of the distal rectum at the level of the puborectalis (*white arrows*) in a male patient on T2-weigted imaging. (*B*) Coronal-oblique view of the pelvis on T2-weighted imaging showing the levator muscle and the anal sphincter. The *arrows* show the oblique course of the levator muscle from the insertion in the fascia of the obturator internus to the top of the anal sphincter.

For efficient planning of the pulse sequences to be employed in MRI, the radiologist should obtain information about the approximate location and size of the tumor, as well as any history of previous surgery or disease of the pelvic organs. Some protocols require cleansing of the rectum with an enema, to eliminate stool residue that might otherwise cause image misinterpretation. However, rectal cleansing is not routinely used in some centers. There is also wide variation on the use of rectal solutions as negative contrast agents against the normal rectal wall on T2-weigted images. Some of the agents commonly used to reduce bowel motion artifacts are glucagon, hyoscyamine, or scopolamine. Rectal MRI is typically performed on a 1.5- or 3-T MRI scanner using a surface pelvic phased-array coil with 4–32 channels. The exam is performed with the patient supine. Anatomic coverage for the localizing sequences extends from the lower level of the kidneys to the perineum. For normal sequences, anatomic coverage extends from the aortic bifurcation to the symphysis of the pubis. For high resolution rectal images, the field of view is centered over the area of the rectum containing the tumor. MRI in most rectal cancer protocols typically include multiplanar T2-weighted (axial, coronal, sagittal, oblique axial, oblique coronal); and multiple axial single b-value diffusion-weighted imaging. Images are obtained with a non-breath-hold turbo spin-echo pulse sequence, featuring a high-resolution matrix, thin section (3 to 5 mm) imaging, and a small (18 to 24 cm) field of view, yielding an in-plane resolution of 0.8 to 1 mm.

MR imaging has excellent anatomical and tissue resolution, but it is unable to distinguish the mucosa from the submucosa of the bowel; these two components are seen as an inner hyperintense layer on T2-weighted imaging. The muscularis propria is visualized as an intermediate hypointense layer, while the mesorectal fat appears hyperintense on T2-weighted imaging. The mesorectal fascia is identified as a thin, low signal intensity layer enveloping the mesorectum and the surrounding perirectal fat (see **Figs. 2** and **3**). Rectal tumors are characterized by intermediate signal intensity—between the high signal intensity of the fat tissue and low signal intensity of the muscular layer—but higher than that of the mucosal and submucosal layers (see

Fig. 5). Rectal cancers typically demonstrate avid enhancement after contrast administration. Adenomatous polyps and superficial T1 tumors are not well visualized by MRI because they do not modify the muscularis propria. Therefore, MRI cannot accurately stage early rectal cancer that does not reach the muscularis propria. T2 tumors are characterized by involvement of the muscular layer, with loss of the interface between the muscle layer and the submucosa. The muscular layer is partially reduced in thickness, although the outer border between the muscularis propria and perirectal fat remains intact. Because of the limitations of MRI in distinguishing between deep T1 and T2 tumors, these are often grouped together as tumors confined to the bowel wall, with smooth margins. The crucial criterion in distinguishing T2 from T3 tumors is extramural spread of the tumor into the perirectal fat, which appears as a rounded or nodular advancing margin or a blurry interface between the muscular layer and the perirectal fat (**Fig. 7**). Extramural spread into the mesorectal fat, measured with MRI imaging, correlates well to histopathological measurements.

Metastatic nodes appear as nodular structures in the mesorectum, usually at or slightly above the level of the tumor, or along the internal iliac or superior rectal vessels. They often have irregular contour and heterogenous signal intensity (see **Figs. 5** and **7**). As mentioned before, size is not an absolute predictor of malignancy, but MRI is more likely to miss nodes smaller than 3 mm in diameter. Similar to ERUS, MRI cannot distinguish between metastatic lymph nodes replaced by tumor and separate extra tumoral deposits in the mesorectum. The use of ultra-small superparamagnetic iron oxide (USPIO) or gadofosveset contrast agents that accumulate, and increase the signal intensity in lymph nodes—seem to facilitate detection of small tumor deposits in enlarged lymph nodes; however, these contrast agents are currently used only in research studies and have not reached the clinic yet. Correlations of MRI images with histological studies have shown that tumor deposits spreading directly off the tumor along the lateral rectal vessels often correspond to extramural vascular invasion (EMVI). The presence of EMVI is an independent predictor of distant metastasis, and a negative prognostic indicator for long-term survival.

When evaluating T3 tumors, one parameter—the minimum distance between the tumor and the mesorectal fascia—is especially significant, as the mesorectal fascia represents the circumferential resection margin (CRM) to be followed during a TME

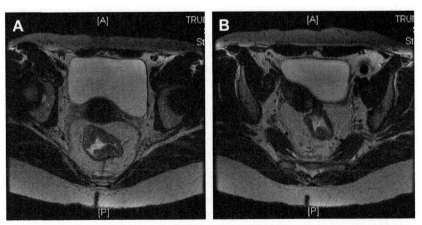

Fig. 7. T2-weighted axial view of a female patient with rectal cancer. The view in (*A*) was obtained at the center of the tumor, while (*B*) was obtained through the upper portion of the tumor. (*B*) shows at least one enlarged mesorectal node highly suspicious for metastasis.

(**Fig. 8**). The distance of the tumor to the CRM is not part of the TNM system, but is nevertheless a strong predictor of tumor recurrence after surgery. Therefore, the distance of the deepest penetration of the tumor into the mesorectal fascia on MRI imaging is commonly used to select treatment and stratify patients for risk of recurrence after TME. In European and Scandinavian countries, the distance of the tumor from the mesorectal fascia is as important as the T or N classification in establishing prognostic groups and directing therapy.

Involvement of the levator muscle or the anal sphincter complex is an important criterion when deciding between an APE or SSP in a patient with a very distal rectal cancer. The funneling of the rectum and the levator muscles towards the anal canal, and the angulation of the lumen of the bowel and surrounding structures at the level of the anorectal ring, limit the usefulness of axial images alone (see **Fig. 2**). Axial images can accurately demonstrate infiltration of a very low rectal cancer into the puborectalis. However, the relationship of the bowel wall to the levators is probably best seen on coronal images (**Fig. 9**).

ERUS

Ultrasound imaging is based on differences in acoustic impedance between tissues. As the different layers of the rectal wall and surrounding tissue have different acoustic impedances, they can be depicted by ultrasound. The resolution of ultrasound depends on the wave length. The 10 mHz crystal commonly used for staging rectal cancer has a resolution of 0.4 mm within a focal range of 1.5 to 4 cm. This level of resolution is sufficient to depict the layers of the bowel wall and to demonstrate other anatomical structures, such as seminal vesicles, prostate, cervix, vagina, blood vessels and perirectal nodes situated within the focal range of the instrument. The puborectalis muscle and the anal sphincters are well visualized on ERUS. However, the levator muscle and other important anatomical structures, such as the fascia propria of the rectum, are not well visualized. The anorectal junction, where the rectal wall funnels towards the anal sphincter, is a particularly difficult area to discern on ERUS imaging because the rectal wall is at an oblique angle in relation to the ultrasound beam. As a result, the layers of the rectal wall tend to appear wider than, but not as

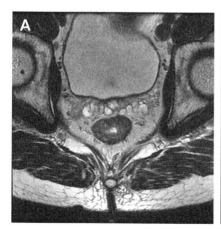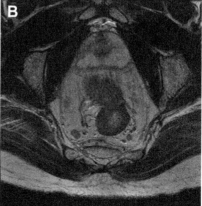

Fig. 8. (*A*) Axial view of a rectal tumor approaching the seminal vesicles. (*B*) Oblique axial view in the same patient showing a right posterior metastatic lymph node close to the mesorectal fascia.

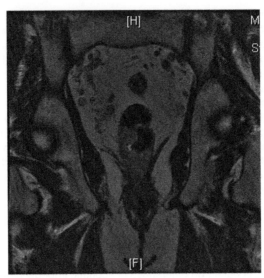

Fig. 9. T2 weighted coronal oblique view of the pelvis in a patient with a low rectal cancer contacting the right levator muscle.

sharp as they appear in other parts of the rectum. Due to the extreme difference in impedance between soft tissue and bone, little transmission occurs through bone because most of the energy is reflected. Bone is usually depicted as a hyperechoic surface with extreme shadowing. However, most pelvic bones are outside the focal range, and only the distal portion of the sacrum is commonly visualized on ERUS.

ERUS is technically challenging and operator dependent. Optimal imaging requires adequate patient preparation and meticulous technique. The rectum should be thoroughly cleansed with an enema immediately before the study. The test is usually performed with the patient positioned in left lateral decubitus, in the knee-chest position. Before inserting the ultrasound probe into the rectum, a digital rectal examination should be performed to identify the location, size, morphology and mobility of the tumor. A proctoscopic exam should always be performed to eliminate stool residue, aspirate air, and avoid shadowing artifacts. It is important to image the entire length of the tumor, as the level of invasion is not uniform along the tumor's length. While the point of deepest penetration is usually located at the center of the tumor, breaks in the submucosa are usually best visualized at the periphery. Furthermore, metastatic lymph nodes are often located at or above the upper margin of the tumor. Therefore, every effort should be made to pass the endorectal probe above the tumor, scanning the entire rectum and mesorectum from the top down. For distal, non-stenotic rectal cancers, the ERUS probe can be inserted into the rectum and blindly advanced beyond the level of the tumor. For higher tumors, the probe should be inserted though a special proctoscope that has already been advanced beyond the tumor.

Optimal visualization of the rectal wall is only possible when the ultrasound probe is at the center of the rectal ampulla, and the water-filled balloon has appropriate acoustic contact with the rectal wall. An eccentric position or inadequate angling of the probe may cause diffraction artifacts and blurry images. Entrapment of air, fecal matter, necrotic tissue or blood clots between the tumor and the water balloon can cause shadowing artifacts that interfere with proper visualization of the rectal wall and adjacent mesorectum. Instillation of the right volume of water in the balloon (usually 30 to 60 mL) is also important because under-inflation can lead to poor contact with the tumor, causing shadowing artifacts, while over-inflation can cause excessive tissue compression and distortion of the anatomy.

The transducer rotates inside the head of the probe to provide a 360° field of view. With the most commonly used probes, the probe is withdrawn manually to scan the entire length of the tumor. With the three-dimensional (3D) automatic acquisition unit, the transducer is automatically moved inward and outward over a distance of 60 mm. Keeping the transducer centered in the lumen of the rectum, as the probe is slowly withdrawn, requires constant adjustment of the position of the transducer to the curvature of the rectum. The automatic withdrawal during 3-D imaging acquisition does not allow the same degree of adjustment as the manual withdrawal of conventional probes; therefore, the quality of the images may vary for different tumors.

Conventional images can be stored either as a single frame or as a movie for later review. 3D automatic acquisition requires special dedicated software that provides a high resolution spatial 3D reconstruction combining a series of closely spaced two-dimensional images. The advantage to 3D ERUS is that the volume can be freely rotated, rendered, tilted and sliced, providing the operator with an infinite variety of section parameters, as well as visualization of the lesion at different angles and in different planes (coronal, frontal, axial). After 3D acquisition, it is possible to select coronal as well as sagittal views immediately. The data can be saved, exported, reviewed and manipulated to derive comprehensive images of the scanned area. Multiplanar reformatting is probably the most useful way to demonstrate the adjacent structures in several planes. With 3D reconstruction, it is then possible to measure tumor size, and evaluate the relationship of tumor to the layers of the bowel wall and the perirectal anatomic structures. In addition, the 3D dataset can be manipulated to render images with enhanced surface features (surface render mode) and depth features (opacity, luminance, thickness and filter settings), further delineating the tumor and its surroundings. On ERUS imaging, rectal tumors appear as expansions of the first hypoechoic layer of the rectal wall, distorting and interrupting the other layers of the rectal wall from the inside out (**Fig. 10**). An ultrasound T classification, similar to the T

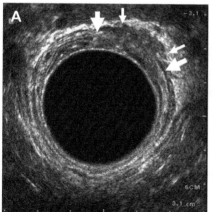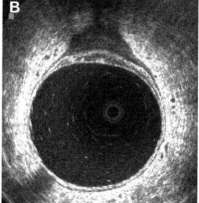

Fig. 10. ERUS image of a rectal cancer (*A*) and an extrarectal tumor infiltrating the muscularis propria from the outside (*B*). The *big arrows* in (*A*) represents the point where the tumor breaks the submucosa, while the *narrow arrows* signals the point where the tumor penetrates though the muscularis propria into the perirectal fat.

classification of the AJCC TNM staging system, is based on tumor disruption of the different echographic layers of the rectal wall (**Fig. 11**). Rectal cancer should be distinguished from extrarectal tumors, which also appear as hypoechoic lesions but invade the layers of the bowel wall from the outside in, often preserving the middle hyperechoic layer that corresponds to the submucosa.

Metastatic lymph nodes appear as hypoechoic deposits, with an echogenicity similar to that of the primary tumor; they are round rather than oval, with discrete or spiculated borders, and are usually found adjacent or proximal to the tumor (see **Fig. 5**). Other features of metastatic lymph nodes are structural inhomogeneity and abnormal hilar echogenicity. Lymph node metastases are easily identified when the entire node is enlarged and replaced by tumor. However, if only a small deposit or micrometastasis is present, the characteristics of the node are unlikely to be sufficiently altered to allow echogenic detection. While some authors consider that

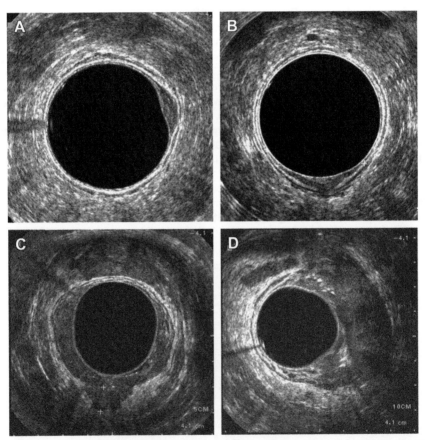

Fig. 11. Endorectal ultrasound images of T1 (*A*), T2 (*B*), T3 (*C*), and T4 (*D*) rectal cancers. The T1 tumor (*A*) is characterized by the partial erosion of the middle hypoechoic layer that corresponds to the submucosa. The T2 tumor (*B*) is characterized by the complete disruption of the submucosa and thickening of the hyperechoic layer that corresponds to the muscularis propria. The T3 tumor (*C*) is characterized by the penetration of the tumor through the muscularis propria and into the perirectal fat. The T4 tumor (*D*) is characterized by the involvement of adjacent organs, in this case the left seminal vesicle.

inflamed, enlarged lymph nodes tend to be hypoechoic and have ill-defined borders, it is difficult to distinguish a neoplastic from an inflammatory node based on echoic appearance. Some ultrasonographers consider any visible mesorectal node to be neoplastic in a patient with a proven rectal cancer. Similar to MRI, ERUS cannot distinguish between mesorectal tumor deposits separated from the primary tumor, and mesorectal lymph nodes totally replaced by tumor.

In experienced hands, ERUS is a very accurate tool for measuring size, circumference and distance of the tumor from various anatomic landmarks (eg, sphincters, prostate, vagina, seminal vesicles, mesorectal fascia, etc). It can also help delineate the relationship of distal rectal cancer from the internal and external sphincter (**Fig. 12**). ERUS can be used to examine the anal sphincters for non-malignant defects as well, helping the surgeon decide whether a sphincter-saving resection is functionally feasible as well as oncologically sound.

DIAGNOSTIC ACCURACY
MRI

There are different criteria for assessing the overall efficacy of the imaging studies used in the preoperative evaluation of rectal cancer. When TNM staging is considered the main criteria for treatment selection and prognostication, the emphasis on the evaluation of imaging studies is based on predicting the T and N classifications (**Fig. 13**). When the treatment decision is based primarily on the probability of having a positive circumferential resection margin with a TME operation, the emphasis on the evaluation of imaging studies is based on assessing the depth of tumor invasion in the bowel wall and the distance of the tumor from the mesorectal fascia (**Fig. 14**). In any case, the determination of the nodal status is always important because the presence of nodal metastasis conveys critical prognostic information, independent of the depth of tumor penetration.

DEPTH OF TUMOR INVASION

Al-Sukhini and colleagues,[1] recently conducted a systematic review and meta-analysis on the diagnostic accuracy of MRI in assessing the depth of tumor invasion, nodal metastasis and CRM. They found significant methodological differences between studies, particularly in the criteria for image interpretation. The reported specificity for depth of tumor invasion was 75% (95% CI 68–80). These results are probably explained by the inherent limitations of MRI imaging. In general, MRI cannot

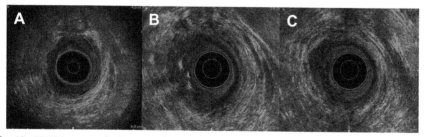

Fig. 12. ERUS images of a low rectal cancer infiltrating the anal sphincter. (*A*) was obtained at the level of the puborectalis, (*B*) at the level of the upper anal canal, and (*C*) at the level of the mid anal canal. The tumor is located in the right side and appears hypoechoic in relation to the surrounding tissues. Notice the very dark hypoechoic ring in images (*B*) and (*C*), interrupted by the tumor. It corresponds to the internal anal sphincter.

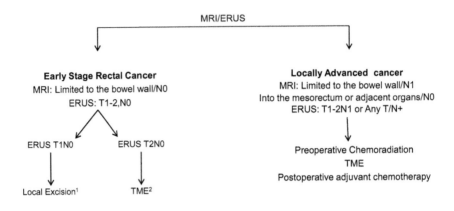

Fig. 13. Treatment algorithm for patients with rectal cancer based on TNM staging.

distinguish between T1 and T2 tumors, and has difficulty distinguishing early T3 tumors from T1/T2 tumors with peritumoral desmoplastic reaction. However, it has a high degree of accuracy in T4 tumors involving adjacent organs (**Fig. 15**).

Endorectal ultrasound has been used to assess the depth of tumor invasion in rectal cancer for almost three decades. Early studies reported a strong correlation between ultrasound images and histopathological analysis. In a review of the raw data from articles published until 1993 on the accuracy and reliability of ERUS in assessing rectal cancer, Solomon et al found an overall correlation of 0.84, with a sensitivity of 0.97, specificity of 0.87%, positive predictive value of 0.97, and negative predictive value of 0. 9.[2] Larger, more recent studies have reported lower correlation. The early high performance of ERUS in staging rectal cancer was probably overestimated due to publication bias.[3] In one of the largest series published so far, the overall agreement

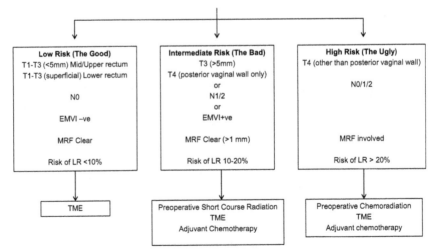

Fig. 14. Treatment algorithm based on MRI imaging. According to this protocol patients are stratified and the treatment selected based on the risk of local recurrence.

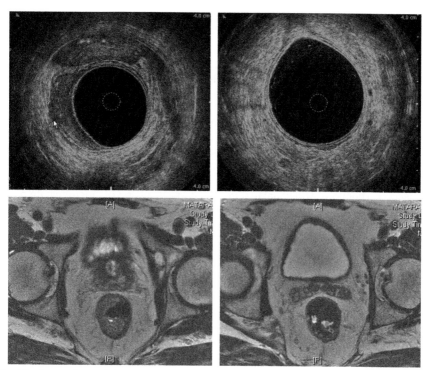

Fig. 15. Comparison of the ERUS and T2-weigted MRI axial images of a rectal cancer in a male patient. The ERUS shows higher anatomical resolution but the MRI provides a wider view of the entire pelvis.

between ERUS and histopathology was 69%, with 18% being overstaged and 13% understaged.[4] There were differences in performance according to the depth of tumor penetration, with the higher performance corresponding to distinguishing between villous adenoma and invasive cancer, and between T1/T2 tumors and T3/T4 tumors. Other series have also reported a high degree of accuracy in identifying tumors localized to the bowel wall.[5]

Because of its ability to depict the layers of the bowel wall, ERUS has been considered particularly useful in the evaluation of early rectal cancer. In our own series, however, the accuracy of ERUS in identifying T1 tumors and distinguishing them from T0 and T2 tumors was only 50%, with an equal number of tumors being overstaged and understaged.[4] This probably reflects the difficulty of demonstrating partial erosion of the middle hyperechoic layer that corresponds to the submucosa, or determining when such erosion is due to tumor invasion or inflammatory or desmoplastic reaction to a villous adenoma. 3D ERUS seems to overcome some of the limitations of conventional ERUS in staging of early rectal cancer. Santoro et al. conducted a prospective study comparing the accuracy of 3D ERUS with high-frequency probe to conventional 2D ERUS in the preoperative staging of early invasive rectal cancer.[6] Reporting on 89 consecutive patients with either rectal villous adenomas (54) or early cancer (35), they found that 3D ERUS was more accurate in identifying both villous adenomas and invasive cancers compared to 2D ultrasound, with accuracy greater than 85% for both T0 and T1 tumors. Kim et al. also reported a higher accuracy for 3D ERUS in identifying T2 tumors (greater than 90% overall), compared to

2D ultrasound.[7] It is possible that tridimensional reconstruction may increase the accuracy of ERUS in staging rectal cancer.

Nodal Metastasis

MRI criteria for diagnosing nodal metastasis has been based on size, with significant differences in opinions regarding the optimal size cutoff for considering a visible lymph node to be metastatic.[8] Some consider that any enlarged perirectal lymph node detected on MRI is metastatic in a patient with known rectal cancer. Others only consider nodes larger than a specific size, usually 5 mm, to be metastatic. However, size alone is an adequate parameter for making a diagnosis of nodal metastasis, as some rectal cancer patients have reactive lymph nodes—particularly after biopsy and other manipulation of the tumors, such as tattooing, that is performed during endoscopy. Therefore, additional features such as spiculated or indeterminate nodal borders and a "mottled heterogeneous" signal are required as criteria in order to call a lymph node metastatic.[8] In N staging, phased-array surface coil provides a larger field of view, including lymph nodes proximal to the tumor, with reported accuracy ranging from 43% to 85%.[1]

ERUS is probably the more accurate modality for detecting nodal metastasis, because it has higher anatomical resolution compared to MRI. It can easily detect nodes as small as 3 mm in greater axis. In general, any hypoechoic round node in the mesorectum, in a patient with a rectal cancer, is considered to be a metastatic lymph node. However, ERUS has the same limitations as MRI in distinguishing metastatic from reactive nodes. In an early series reported by Solomon, the correlation between ERUS and histopathology in assessing nodal metastasis was only 0.58, with a sensitivity of 0.79, specificity of 0.80, positive predictive value of 0.74 and negative predictive value of 0.84.[2] In our series, the accuracy of ERUS in diagnosing nodal metastasis was 64%.[4]

Although most metastatic nodes are located in the vicinity of the tumor, ERUS has a very short focal range and can easily miss lymph nodes located farther away from the tumor, particularly in tumors located in the upper rectum. ERUS cannot detect lymph nodes located in the pelvic sidewalls along the branches of the internal iliac vessels.

MESORECTAL FASCIA

The discovery that neoplastic involvement of the CRM is one of the most important predictors of local relapse in rectal cancer patients treated with TME, along with the possibility of identifying the mesorectal fascia—the natural plane of dissection in TME surgery—on thin slicing MRI, added a new dimension to the MRI imaging of rectal cancer patients.[9,10] Over the last 15 years, assessment of the distance of the tumor to the mesorectal fascia has became one of the most important parameters in the preoperative evaluation of rectal cancer patients, particularly when short-course preoperative radiation has not been used for all tumors extending beyond the muscularis propria. Beets-Tan et al reported high accuracy and consistency of MRI in predicting a tumor-free resection, in a series of 76 patients treated with TME.[9] Other studies later confirmed these results.[11] The MERCURY study, a prospective observational study assessing the accuracy of MRI in predicting a curative resection in rectal cancer, reported 92% specificity in predicting a clear resection margin.[12] A recent systematic review and meta-analysis has found that MRI had a sensitivity of 77% (95% CI, 57%-90%) and specificity of 94% (95% CI 88%–97%) in predicting CRM involvement. MRI was more specific for CRM involvement than for T category, but the sensitivity of both elements was not significantly different.[1]

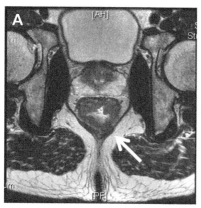
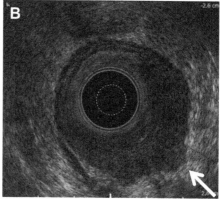

Fig. 16. MRI and ERUS image of a tumor infiltrating the levator muscle. An axial T2-weighted MRI (*A*) of a low rectal cancer reaching the left posterior aspect of the levator muscle. ERUS (*B*) of the same tumor showing infiltration of the levator muscle. The *arrows* point to the area where the tumor infiltrates the levator muscle.

The clinical relevance of the MRI assessment of rectal cancer was heightened by the extended follow-up of the patients entered in the MERCURY trial. The investigators reported that MRI was able to identify a group of rectal cancer patients with good prognosis (clear CRM, no evidence of extramural vascular invasion, T2 or T3 <5 mm and not involving the intersphincteric plane), with 3% local recurrence and 85% 5-year disease-free survival after treatment with surgery alone.[13]

Endorectal ultrasound can easily identify the CRM at the level of the seminal vesicles, the prostate and vagina, but it cannot reliably depict the MRF, particularly in the posterior aspect of the mesorectum (**Figs. 16** and **17**). One study has reported a good correlation between ERUS and MRI imaging in predicting margin involvement, in a series of 52 patients with locally advanced rectal cancer. However, patients in this study were treated with neoadjuvant therapy, and the correlation to the histopathological measurement of the closest radial margin was low for both ERUS and MRI.[14]

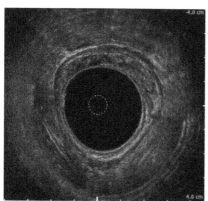
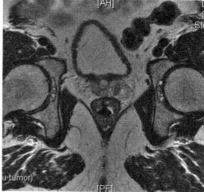

Fig. 17. Comparison of the ERUS and T2-weigted MRI oblique coronal images of a distal early stage rectal cancer in a male patient. The ERUS shows in more detail the layers of the bowel wall and the relationship of the tumor to the prostate, compared to the MRI image.

Table 1
Comparison between MRI and ERUS in evaluation of patients with rectal cancer

	MRI	ERUS
Availability	Radiology department	Doctor's office
Patient contraindications	Pacemaker Metal implants Claustrophobia	None
Anatomic resolution	Good	Excellent
Tissue resolution	Excellent (potentially improved by contrast, DWI, DCE)	Good
Anatomic coverage	Wide	Narrow
Operator dependency	High	Very high
Early cancers (T1s vs. T1 vs. T2)	Poor	Good
T1/T2 vs. T3	Good	Good
T4	Excellent	Only anterior tumors
Mesorectal nodes	Moderate	Moderate
Internal iliac/superior rectal nodes	Good	Poor
Relationship to mesorectal fascia	Excellent	Poor
Infiltration of levator muscle	Good	Moderate
Infiltration of anal sphincter	Moderate	Good

In summary, many case series, and several reviews and meta-analyses, have compared the diagnostic performance of MRI and ERUS in the pre-treatment staging of rectal cancer. The results are variable and difficult to reconcile, due to changes in imaging technology over time, variation in imaging interpretation criteria and reference standards, and patient selection. However, they do allow us to draw some conclusions regarding the diagnostic performance of each of these imaging modalities for different tumor characteristics that are important in the preoperative evaluation of rectal cancer (**Table 1**).

ASSESSING TUMOR RESPONSE

The accuracy of MRI and ERUS in restaging rectal cancer after neoadjuvant chemoradiotherapy is disappointing. Both MRI and ERUS are limited by an inability to differentiate residual tumor from radiation-induced edema, inflammation, or fibrosis. Vanagunas and colleagues[15] found that ERUS showed an accuracy of only 48% in determining T stage after chemoradiation therapy; in their study, 38% of lesions were overstaged and 14% were understaged. Mezzi and colleagues[16] found that, after neoadjuvant chemoradiation, ERUS and MRI correctly determined the T stage in 46% and 44% of tumors, compared to the histologic T stage. The percentages were higher for both ERUS and MRI when nodal involvement was considered: 69% and 62%, respectively. ERUS was superior to MRI in identifying patients with T0 to T2 tumors (44% vs 33%, $P>.05$) and N0 disease (87% vs 52%, $P = .013$). However, MRI was more accurate than ERUS in T and N staging of patients with advanced disease after radiotherapy (T3–T4: 52% vs 48%, N1– N2: 75% vs 48%, respectively), although the differences did not reach statistical significance.[16] Tumor restaging after neoadjuvant therapy remains problematic, and it is hoped that a combination of new MRI sequences, such as diffusion weighted (DW) MRI, and functional imaging with positron emission tomography (PET) may improve accuracy.

REFERENCES

1. Al Sukhni E, Milot L, Fruitman M, et al. Diagnostic accuracy of MRI for assessment of T category, lymph node metastases, and circumferential resection margin involvement in patients with rectal cancer: a systematic review and meta-analysis. Ann Surg Oncol 2012;19:2212–23.
2. Solomon MJ, McLeod RS. Endoluminal transrectal ultrasonography: accuracy, reliability, and validity. Dis Colon Rectum 1993;36(2):200–5.
3. Harewood GC. Assessment of publication bias in the reporting of EUS performance in staging rectal cancer. Am J Gastroenterol 2005;100:808–16.
4. Garcia-Aguilar J, Pollack J, Lee SH, et al. Accuracy of endorectal ultrasonography in preoperative staging of rectal tumors. Dis Colon Rectum 2002;45(1):10–5.
5. Sailer M, Leppert R, Kraemer M, et al. The value of endorectal ultrasound in the assessment of adenomas, T1- and T2-carcinomas. Int J Colorectal Dis 1997;12: 214–9.
6. Santoro GA, BED, Di Falco G. Three dimensional endorectal ultrasonography in the evaluation of early invasive rectal cancer. Colorectal Dis 2004;6(Suppl 2): 1–34.
7. Kim JC, Cho YK, Kim SY, et al. Comparative study of three-dimensional and conventional endorectal ultrasonography used in rectal cancer staging. Surg Endosc 2002;16(9):1280–5.
8. Kim JH, Beets GL, Kim MJ, et al. High-resolution MR imaging for nodal staging in rectal cancer: are there any criteria in addition to the size? Eur J Radiol 2004; 52(1):78–83.
9. Beets-Tan RG, Beets GL, Vliegen RF, et al. Accuracy of magnetic resonance imaging in prediction of tumour-free resection margin in rectal cancer surgery. Lancet 2001;357(9255):497–504.
10. Brown G, Richards CJ, Newcombe RG, et al. Rectal carcinoma: thin-section MR imaging for staging in 28 patients. Radiology 1999;211(1):215–22.
11. Lahaye MJ, Engelen SM, Nelemans PJ, et al. Imaging for predicting the risk factors–the circumferential resection margin and nodal disease–of local recurrence in rectal cancer: a meta-analysis. Semin Ultrasound CT MRI 2005;26(4):259–68.
12. MERCURY Study Group. Diagnostic accuracy of preoperative magnetic resonance imaging in predicting curative resection of rectal cancer: prospective observational study. BMJ 2006;333(7572):779.
13. Taylor FG, Quirke P, Heald RJ, et al. Preoperative high-resolution magnetic resonance imaging can identify good prognosis stage I, II, and III rectal cancer best managed by surgery alone. Ann Surg 2011;253(4):711–9.
14. Phang PT, Gollub MJ, Loh BD, et al. Accuracy of endorectal ultrasound for measurement of the closest predicted radial mesorectal margin for rectal cancer. Dis Colon Rectum 2012;55(1):59–64.
15. Vanagunas A, Lin DE, Stryker SJ. Accuracy of endoscopic ultrasound for restaging rectal cancer following neoadjuvant chemoradiation therapy. Am J Gastroenterol 2004;99(1):109–12.
16. Mezzi G, Arcidiacono PG, Carrara S, et al. Endoscopic ultrasound and magnetic resonance imaging for restagingrectal cancer after radiotherapy. World J Gastroenterol 2009;15(44):5563–7.

Current Controversies in Neoadjuvant Chemoradiation of Rectal Cancer

P. Terry Phang, MD, MSc, FRCSC[a],*, Xiaodong Wang, MD[b]

KEYWORDS

- Rectal cancer • Neo-adjuvant chemoradiation • Short course • Long course
- Complete pathologic response

KEY POINTS

- Total mesorectal excision with preoperative radiation and chemotherapy provide the lowest local recurrence rates for rectal cancer.
- Timing of surgery after preoperative chemoradiation is being increased to optimize tumor downstaging.
- Permissive observation of complete clinical response is investigational at present.
- Preoperative and postoperative radiation provides improved local cancer control for superficial cancers removed by local excision.
- Good prognostic tumor characteristics are being investigated with the aim of selecting patients for whom preoperative radiation may be avoided.

BACKGROUND

In the history of rectal cancer surgery, outcomes have previously been less favorable than for colon cancer, with local recurrence rates on the order of 25% versus 5% and 5-year survival rates on the order of 30% versus 50%. To improve on rectal cancer surgery outcomes, postoperative (adjuvant) combination radiation and chemotherapy regimens were recommended, based on trials conducted by the US North Central Cancer Treatment Group (NCCTG),[1] the Gastrointestinal Tumor Study Group (GITSG),[2] and the National Surgical Adjuvant Breast and Bowel Project (NSABP).[3] However, outcomes of rectal cancer remained less favorable despite this standard adjuvant treatment.[4]

A remarkable improvement in outcomes of rectal cancer was reported by Heald and Ryall[5] using the technique of total mesorectal excision (TME). The report on Heald's surgical results without adjuvant treatments by MacFarlane and colleagues[6] showed

[a] Department of Surgery, St. Paul's Hospital, University of British Columbia, 1081 Burrard Street, Vancouver, BC V6Z 1Y6, Canada; [b] Gastrointestinal Surgery Centre, West China Hospital, Sichuan University, No. 37 Guo Xue Xiang, Chengdu, Sichuan 610041, China
* Corresponding author.
E-mail address: tphang@providencehealth.bc.ca

Surg Oncol Clin N Am 23 (2014) 79–92
http://dx.doi.org/10.1016/j.soc.2013.09.008
1055-3207/14/$ – see front matter © 2014 Elsevier Inc. All rights reserved.

local recurrence outcomes to be superior to non-TME surgery with adjuvant treatments, 7% versus 19%.

The second remarkable improvement in outcomes of rectal cancer was preoperative (neoadjuvant) radiation, introduced in the Swedish rectal cancer trials.[7] Local recurrence and survival were improved in a randomized trial using short-course preoperative radiation versus surgery alone. However, surgery in this study was not based on TME technique. Outcomes with short-course preoperative radiation plus non-TME surgery remained suboptimal, stressing the importance of TME surgery as the main standard treatment of rectal cancer.

The first randomized trial using TME was reported by Dutch investigators,[8] who demonstrated that TME surgery could be learned and adopted by general surgeons, with good results. Norway has also adopted TME surgery on a national basis, with national local recurrence rates of 8%.[9] Furthermore, the main finding of the Dutch trial was that the combination of short-course preoperative radiation plus TME had the lowest local recurrence rate.[10] This large multicenter study provided new outcomes standards for rectal cancer that approach outcomes for colon cancer.[11] The protocol of preoperative short-course radiation and TME surgery has also been used for populations in Sweden, Denmark, and British Columbia in Canada.[10–12]

Preoperative radiation was demonstrated to be superior to postoperative radiation in a German randomized trial,[13] which also used TME as the standard surgery technique. Preoperative radiation reduced local recurrence by half compared with postoperative radiation (6% vs 13%). Moreover, the downstaging effect of preoperative radiation resulted in increased sphincter-preserving resection with less permanent colostomies in patients preoperatively judged to require abdominoperineal resection (39% vs 19%). This sphincter-preserving effect from downstaging by preoperative long-course chemoradiation was also seen in a Korean trial.[14] The NSABP also conducted a trial of preoperative versus postoperative chemoradiation. Though unable to complete its full study because of incomplete recruitment, the NSABP did report trends toward improved disease-free survival with preoperative treatments, 64% versus 52% at 7 years.[15]

On this basis, preoperative radiation combined with chemotherapy has been adopted as the standard protocol for rectal cancer management by the National Institutes of Health (NIH) and the National Comprehensive Cancer Network (NCCN) in the United States and Canada.

CONTROVERSIES: OUTLINE

The evolution of the management of rectal cancer provides a background for controversies over preoperative radiation in current management. Controversies to be discussed here include:

- The protocol of preoperative radiation (short vs long course): efficacy and toxicity
- Whether chemotherapy is used in combination with radiation, and which chemotherapy drugs are used
- The optimum timing of surgery after radiation to achieve maximum downstaging
- Whether radiation is used for all rectal cancers or on a selected basis only
- The preferred radiation protocol for treating superficial rectal cancer being considered for local excision
- Whether endocavitary radiation can be used as an effective treatment

Table 1 lists randomized trials for each of the topics.

THE PROTOCOL OF PREOPERATIVE RADIATION: EFFICACY AND TOXICITY

Two randomized trials have compared short-course and long-course preoperative chemoradiation. In the Polish trial,[16] there was no difference in local recurrence or survival between short-course and long-course preoperative chemoradiation. Of note, there was a trend toward lower local recurrence with short-course preoperative radiation. In addition, although downstaging after long-course preoperative chemoradiation should facilitate sphincter-preserving resection, there was no difference in rates of abdominoperineal resection between short-course and long-course preoperative radiation groups. A second randomized trial that compared short-course with long-course preoperative chemoradiation has been reported from the Trans-Tasman group.[17] Again, there was no difference in local recurrence or survival between groups. The investigators suggested that long-course preoperative chemoradiation may have nonsignificant benefit for local recurrence of distal rectal cancers less than 5 cm from the anus.

Toxicity of short-course preoperative radiation is predicted to be lower than for long-course preoperative chemoradiation, owing to its lower radiobiological equivalent effect. Although larger fraction size used in short-course radiation is associated with higher risk for late toxicity, no difference in late toxicity was reported in the 2 trials that compared short-course and long-course preoperative radiation.[17,18] Of note, the Swedish rectal cancer study using short-course preoperative radiation did report increased toxicity with femoral fractures, thromboembolism, small-bowel obstruction, and postoperative mortality.[19,20] The increased toxicity in the initial Swedish trials was accounted for by use of extended radiation fields up to L1, use of 2 rather than 4 portals, and absence of blocking. With the use of small radiation fields, 4 portals, and blocking in the Polish study, toxicity was less for short-course preoperative radiation in the acute phase, and equivalent in the late phase relative to long-course preoperative chemoradiation.[16]

The German trial showed that toxicity was reduced with chemoradiation given preoperatively versus postoperatively, 27% versus 40% in the early stage and 14% versus 24% in the late stage.[13] The reduced toxicity resulted in more patients completing the full dose of chemoradiation in the preoperative group, which in part may account for the improved outcomes seen with preoperative treatments. In the Polish trial, 98% of patients completed the prescribed short-course radiation treatment, compared with 69% of patients completing the prescribed long-course treatments.[17]

Intensity-modulated arc therapy has been used to minimize small-bowel radiation toxicity. Radiation is delivered in 3 to 6 arcs for a 180 cGy fraction while lowering total small-bowel dose from 17.0 Gy to 12.4 Gy and, hence, small-bowel toxicity.[21–24] However, a phase II study reported in abstract form found no difference in gastrointestinal toxicity, 51% versus 58%, on comparing intensity-modulated with conventional preoperative chemoradiation, and showed a pathologic complete response of 15%.[25]

Pelvic radiation has adverse effects on the bowel, bladder, and sexual function. Impairments occur more with postoperative than with preoperative radiation.[13] However, there was no difference in bowel impairment between preoperative short-course versus long-course radiation with respect to incontinence (72% vs 65%) or stool frequency (4 vs 5).[17] Bladder incontinence occurs in about 40%, and sexual dysfunction in about 30% of irradiated patients who undergo rectal cancer surgery.[26,27]

WHETHER CHEMOTHERAPY IS USED IN COMBINATION WITH RADIATION AND WHICH CHEMOTHERAPY DRUGS ARE USED

The rationale for using a combination of chemotherapy and radiation is based on adjuvant studies by the NCCTG, GITSG, and NSABP between 1980 and 1990.[1–4] After

Table 1
Randomized trials for each of the topics

Topic	Study	Groups	Follow-Up (mo)	Local Recurrence	Survival
The protocol of preoperative radiation-efficacy and toxicity	Swedish Rectal Cancer Trial,[7] 1997	Preoperative radiotherapy + surgery vs Surgery	75	11% vs 27%, $P<.001$	OS (58% vs 48%, $P = .004$)
	Kapiteijn et al,[8] 2001	Preoperative radiotherapy + TME vs TME	24.9	2.4% vs 8.2%, $P<.001$	OS (82% vs 81.8%, $P = .84$)
	Sauer et al,[13] 2004	Preoperative chemoradiation vs postoperative chemoradiation	46	6% vs 13%, $P = .006$	OS (76% vs 74%, $P = .80$) DFS (68% vs 65%, $P = .32$)
	Roh et al,[15] 2009	Preoperative chemoradiation vs postoperative chemoradiation	72	10.7% vs 10.7%, $P = .693$	OS (74.5% vs 65.6%, $P = .065$) DFS (64.7% vs 53.4%, $P = .011$)
	Bujko et al,[16] 2006	Short-course preoperative radiotherapy vs Long-course chemoradiation	48	9.0% vs 14.2%, $P = .170$	OS (67.2% vs 66.2%, $P = .960$) DFS (58.4% vs 55.6%, $P = .820$)
	Ngan et al,[17] 2012	Short-course preoperative chemoradiation vs Long-course preoperative chemoradiation	70	7.5% vs 4.4%, $P = .24$	OS (74% vs 70%, $P = .62$)
Whether chemotherapy is used in combination with radiation and which chemotherapy drugs are used	Gerard et al,[30] 2006	Preoperative radiotherapy + chemotherapy vs Preoperative radiotherapy	81	8.1% vs 16.5%, $P = .004$	OS (67.5% vs 67.9%, $P = .684$) DFS (59.4% vs 55.5%)
	Bosset et al,[31] 2006	Preoperative radiotherapy vs Preoperative chemoradiation vs Preoperative radiotherapy + postoperative chemoradiation vs Preoperative chemoradiation + postoperative chemoradiation	64.8	17.1% vs 8.7% vs 9.6% vs 7.6%, $P = .002$	OS (preoperative radiotherapy 65.8% vs preoperative chemoradiation 64.8%, $P = .84$; postoperative chemoradiation 67.2% vs no postoperative chemoradiation 63.2%, $P = .12$) DFS (preoperative radiotherapy 54.4% vs preoperative chemoradiation 56.1%, $P = .52$; postoperative chemoradiation 52.2% vs no postoperative chemoradiation 58.2%, $P = .13$)
	Hofheinz et al,[33] 2012	Postoperative radiotherapy + capecitabine vs + fluorouracil	52	6% vs 7%, $P = .67$	OS (81% vs 71%, $P = .05$) DFS (75% vs 67%, $P = .07$)

The optimum timing of surgery after radiation to achieve maximum downstaging	Habr-Gama et al,[49] 2010	Surgery vs nonoperative treatment	57.3	Surgery: 9%	OS (88% vs 97%, P = .01) DFS (83% vs 84%, P = .09)
Whether radiation is used for all rectal cancers or on a selected basis only	Peeters et al,[57] 2007	Preoperative radiotherapy + TME vs TME	73.2	5.6% vs 10.9%, P<.001	OS (64.2% vs 63.5%, P = .902)
	Sebag-Montefiore et al,[58] 2009	Preoperative radiotherapy vs postoperative chemoradiotherapy	48	4.4% vs 10.6%, P<.0001	OS (P = .40) DFS (77.5% vs 71.5%, P = .013)
The preferred radiation protocol for treating superficial rectal cancer being considered for local excision	Chakravarti et al,[68] 1999	Local resection + postoperative irradiation vs local resection	60	Local control rate 72% vs 90%, P = .18	Not reported

Abbreviations: DFS, disease-free survival; OS, overall survival.

rectal cancer surgery, patients were randomized to receive 5-fluorouracil–based chemotherapy plus radiation or radiation alone. The chemoradiation treatment groups had a decrease in local recurrence (by 46%) and increased survival (by 29%) compared with radiation-alone groups.

Chemotherapy increases early-phase toxicity (nausea, vomiting, diarrhea, stomatitis, leukopenia, thrombocytopenia) in comparison with radiation alone, but does not increase late-phase toxicity. Methyl-CCNU was discontinued from the regimens because of excessive toxicity.[28] Levamisole and leucovorin were shown to further improve the effectiveness of 5-fluorouracil in reducing metastatic disease without increasing toxicity.[29]

Chemoradiation has been shown to improve local recurrence in comparison with radiation alone in the preoperative setting, 8% versus 17%.[30,31]

More recently, capecitabine, the oral form of 5-fluorouracil, has replaced intravenous 5-fluorouracil and leucovorin as the chemotherapy drug used with preoperative long-course radiation. With capecitabine, overall clinical downstaging response rate was 57% and complete pathologic response rate was 24%, similar to response rates using intravenous 5-fluorouracil.[32] Toxicity with capecitabine and radiation was similar to toxicity with intravenous 5-fluorouracil and leucovorin. Furthermore, capecitabine with preoperative radiation was associated with improved disease-free survival at 3 years in comparison with infused 5-fluoruracil, 76% versus 67%.[33]

Addition of irinotecan or oxaliplatin to capecitabine and radiation preoperatively did not significantly increase overall downstaging, at about 60%.[34–37] Addition of bevacizumab (antiangiogenic) or cetuximab (epidermal growth factor receptor inhibitor) to capecitabine and radiation preoperatively also did not significantly increase overall downstaging.[38–40]

To summarize, chemotherapy added to radiation improves local recurrence rates in both preoperative and postoperative settings. The current recommended chemotherapy for use with preoperative radiation is capecitabine.

THE OPTIMUM TIMING OF SURGERY AFTER RADIATION TO ACHIEVE MAXIMUM DOWNSTAGING

As discussed in the previous section, use of preoperative long-course chemoradiation was not superior to preoperative short-course radiation with respect to local control, rate of sphincter-preserving surgery, or toxicity. However, clear advantages of preoperative long-course chemoradiation are (1) the use of the downstaging response for prognosis and (2) guiding management considerations of permissive observation, so-called watch and wait, or further preoperative chemotherapy in the setting of a complete clinical response. By contrast, downstaging after short-course preoperative radiation when surgery is performed in the week following radiation is minimal, but more significant downstaging is observed when surgery is delayed for more than 10 days after radiation.[41,42] Downstaging has been reported with delay in surgery for 6 weeks after completion of short-course preoperative radiation, but to a lesser extent in comparison with long-course chemoradiation.[43,44] Data on downstaging after short-course radiation is pending from a prospective Swedish trial in which the interval to surgery was varied.[45]

Preoperative chemoradiation in the German trial demonstrated the prognostic value of assessing tumor response. Five-year disease-free survival was 86% for complete pathologic response, 75% for tumor regression of 25% to 75%, and 63% for tumor regression of less than 25%.[46] An Italian study also reported excellent outcomes for cases of complete pathologic response with 5-year disease-free survival of 85%,

2% local recurrence, and 9% distant metastases.[47] A pooled analysis of pathologic complete response in 27 articles reported 5-year disease-free survival of 83%.[48]

Permissive observation of complete clinical response has been studied by Habr-Gama and colleagues[49,50] in a study comparing surgery with observation. Complete clinical response after preoperative chemoradiation using 5-fluorouracil and leucovorin was observed in 27% of patients; permissive observation in these patients resulted in 5-year disease-free survival of 92%. In this study, patients with partial clinical response underwent surgery. Of surgical patients demonstrating complete pathologic response, 5-year disease-free survival was 83%. Habr-Gama's group assesses response at 10 weeks following chemoradiation, and permissive observation is recommended for patients with a complete clinical response. Others have reported that complete pathologic response was associated with incomplete clinical response and residual mucosal abnormality in 54% of cases.[51] Further prospective data are needed before the approach of permissive observation can be generally adopted.[52]

In a strategy to increase complete clinical response, additional preoperative chemotherapy before or after preoperative chemoradiation is being investigated.[53,54]

In summary, the optimum interval between preoperative radiation and surgery has not been defined. Complications are minimized if surgery is performed in the first week or 4 to 8 weeks after radiation when the inflammatory response to radiation is less. It is currently suggested that the optimum interval within which to assess for complete clinical response is 10 to 12 weeks after chemoradiation.

WHETHER RADIATION IS USED FOR ALL RECTAL CANCERS OR ON A SELECTED BASIS ONLY

Current NCCN and NIH guidelines used in the United States and Canada recommend use of preoperative chemoradiation for stage 2 and 3 rectal cancers.[55,56] The Dutch TME and United Kingdom CR07 trials both showed improved local recurrence from use of preoperative short-course radiation over TME surgery alone.[57,58]

Nevertheless, TME surgery without preoperative radiation can result in acceptable local recurrence rates of less than 10% and survival rates equivalent to preoperative radiation plus TME surgery.[57] Also of note is that preoperative radiation was not beneficial for upper-third rectal cancers in the Dutch trial. Retrospective studies have demonstrated low local recurrence rates for selected T3N0 rectal cancers treated with surgery alone.[59–64] Heald and colleagues[65] reported use of prognostic magnetic resonance imaging (MRI) features to select patients for use or avoidance of preoperative chemoradiation. Prognostic MRI features used to select patients for no preoperative chemoradiation included cancer less than 5 mm beyond the muscularis propria, mesorectal fascia more than 1 mm from the advancing edge of the tumor, and absence of extramural vascular invasion; mesorectal nodes were not used as an indication for preoperative chemoradiation. The multicenter, multinational MERCURY study group reported that with these MRI criteria, patients treated with surgery alone had a local recurrence rate of 3% and a 5-year survival rate of 85%.[66]

In summary, good prognosis features include location in the upper third and predicted clear circumferential resection margins. Poor prognosis features include distal location, involved mesorectal fascia, vascular invasion, and extramesorectal lymphadenopathy. In the absence of involved mesorectal fascia, mesorectal lymphadenopathy does not infer poor prognosis for local control when TME surgery is performed. Further study is required to confirm that preoperative radiation is not required for rectal cancer demonstrating good preoperative features.

THE PREFERRED RADIATION PROTOCOL FOR TREATING SUPERFICIAL RECTAL CANCER BEING CONSIDERED FOR LOCAL EXCISION

For clinically node-negative disease, local excision has been considered for smaller lesions as an alternative to radical surgery. Radiation after local excision of superficial cancers resulted in local control in 78% to 90% and 5-year survival of 74% to 88%.[67–69] Local excision alone for T1 lesions and local excision followed by postoperative chemoradiation for T2 lesions resulted in local recurrence and 10-year survival of 8% and 18% and 84% and 66%, respectively.[70] Although functional outcomes are excellent, the oncologic outcomes of local excision are significantly inferior to those of radical surgery for T1 and T2 rectal cancers, whereby local control and 5-year survival are in the range of 95% and 90%, respectively.

An alternative strategy for superficial cancers is preoperative radiation. As discussed earlier, there is substantial downstaging of most tumors and a 10% to 25% complete clinical response rate. Previous studies have reported outcomes for preoperative chemoradiation followed by transanal excision not using transanal endoscopic microsurgery (TEM).[71–73] Local recurrence was 0% for ypT0 (complete clinical response), 0% to 6% for ypT1, and 6% to 20% for ypT2. Five-year disease-free survival was 67% to 93% depending on whether there was complete pathologic response in the local excision specimens. Wound complications after local excision are higher with preoperative chemoradiation, 26% versus 0% for no preoperative radiation.[74,75] Major wound separation requiring additional surgery occurred in 9% of patients.

These results from a relatively small number of patients using preoperative chemoradiation and local excision provide a basis for further study. TEM may improve local recurrence over the traditional transanal excision technique.[76] The CARTS trial of preoperative long-course chemoradiation followed by local excision using TEM techniques is currently enrolling patients.[77]

WHETHER ENDOCAVITARY RADIATION CAN BE USED AS EFFECTIVE TREATMENT

Endocavitary radiation has been used for superficial rectal cancers, with local control of 79% to 83% and survival of 65% to 84% at 5 years.[78–81] Local control was improved with mobility of the lesion and T1 versus T2 depth of invasion. In another study, endocavitary radiation resulted in local control of 100% of T1 lesions and 85% of mobile T2 lesions.[82] Toxicity from endocavitary radiation with 60 to 190 Gy in 2 to 5 fractions was seen in 80% of patients. However, patients who are poor surgical candidates tolerate this treatment without loss of sphincter function.

Salvage abdominoperineal resection after failed endocavitary radiation results in 5-year disease-specific survival of 66% to 87%.[80,83] However, salvage surgery in these patients was associated with high rates of tumor perforation, injury to genitourinary organs, and delayed wound healing.

Endocavitary radiation given preoperatively for T3 to T4 cancers has undergone preliminary study, with 5-year local recurrence of 5% and disease-free survival of 65%.[84,85] Toxicity from the treatment dose of 26 Gy in 4 fractions was favorable, with grade 2 proctitis observed in all patients. A randomized trial is planned to compare preoperative high dose endocavitary radiation with external-beam radiation and chemotherapy.

SUMMARY

Preoperative radiation with concurrent capecitabine results in maximum downstaging, and is the protocol currently recommended for management of stage 2 and 3 rectal cancer in the United States and Canada (NCCN, NIH). Short-course preoperative radiation results in local recurrence and sphincter-preserving resection rates equivalent to those for long-course preoperative chemoradiation. Sweden and the Netherlands routinely use short-course preoperative radiation as their preferred protocol. Recommendations for preoperative chemoradiation and short-course radiation are based on randomized trials data, and are preferred over postoperative radiation.

With complete clinical response to preoperative chemoradiation, there are limited data on the efficacy of permissive observation. Prospective evaluation of permissive observation has begun in multiple centers worldwide. The optimal interval between the completion of radiation and operation and the role and timing of additional preoperative chemotherapy are being investigated.

Bowel dysfunction resulting from preoperative radiation and TME surgery is problematic. A prospective study in the United Kingdom is evaluating TME without preoperative radiation for good-risk T3 lesions irrespective of nodal appearance.

Local excision using the TEM technique after chemoradiation results in less bowel dysfunction in comparison with TME, and this option is being investigated prospectively for small residual lesions. Preoperative endocavitary radiation is also being prospectively investigated.

REFERENCES

1. Krook JE, Moertel CG, Gunderson LL, et al. Effective surgical adjuvant therapy for high risk rectal carcinoma. N Engl J Med 1991;324:709–15.
2. Gastrointestinal Tumor Study Group. Prolongation of disease free interval in surgically treated rectal carcinoma. N Engl J Med 1985;312:1465–72.
3. Fisher B, Wolmark N, Rockette H, et al. Postoperative adjuvant chemotherapy or radiation therapy for rectal cancer: results from NSABP protocol R-01. J Natl Cancer Inst 1988;80:21–9.
4. NIH consensus conference on adjuvant therapy for patients with colon and rectal cancer. JAMA 1990;264:1444–50.
5. Heald RJ, Ryall RD. Recurrence and survival after total mesorectal excision for rectal cancer. Lancet 1986;1:1479–82.
6. MacFarlane JK, Ryall RD, Heald RJ. Mesorectal excision for rectal cancer. Lancet 1993;341(8843):457–60.
7. Swedish Rectal Cancer Trial. Improved survival with preoperative radiotherapy in resectable rectal cancer. N Engl J Med 1997;336(14):980–7.
8. Kapiteijn E, Marijnen CA, Nagtegaal ID, et al, Dutch Colorectal Cancer Group. Preoperative radiotherapy combined with total mesorectal excision for resectable rectal cancer. N Engl J Med 2001;345(9):638–46.
9. Wibe A, Møller B, Norstein J, et al, Norwegian Rectal Cancer Group. A national strategic change in treatment policy for rectal cancer–implementation of total mesorectal excision as routine treatment in Norway. A national audit. Dis Colon Rectum 2002;45(7):857–66.
10. Bülow S, Harling H, Iversen LH, et al, Danish Colorectal Cancer Group. Improved survival after rectal cancer in Denmark. Colorectal Dis 2010;12(7 Online):e37–42. http://dx.doi.org/10.1111/j.1463-1318.2009.02012.x.
11. Birgisson H, Talbäck M, Gunnarsson U, et al. Improved survival in cancer of the colon and rectum in Sweden. Eur J Surg Oncol 2005;31(8):845–53.
12. Phang PT, McGahan CE, McGregor G, et al. Effects of change in rectal cancer management on outcomes in British Columbia. Can J Surg 2010;53:225–31.

13. Sauer R, Becker H, Hohenberger W, et al, German Rectal Cancer Study Group. Preoperative versus postoperative chemoradiotherapy for rectal cancer. N Engl J Med 2004;351:1731–40.

14. Park JH, Kim JH, Ahn SD, et al. Prospective phase II study of preoperative chemoradiation with capecitabine in locally advanced rectal cancer. Cancer Res Treat 2004;36(6):354–9. http://dx.doi.org/10.4143/crt.2004.36.6.354.

15. Roh MS, Colangelo LH, O'Connell MJ, et al. Preoperative multimodality therapy improves disease-free survival in patients with carcinoma of the rectum: NSABP R-03. J Clin Oncol 2009;27(31):5124–30. http://dx.doi.org/10.1200/JCO.2009.22.0467.

16. Bujko K, Nowacki MP, Nasierowska-Guttmejer A, et al. Long-term results of a randomized trial comparing preoperative short-course radiotherapy with preoperative conventionally fractionated chemoradiation for rectal cancer. Br J Surg 2006;93:1215–23.

17. Ngan SY, Burmeister B, Fisher RJ, et al. Randomized trial of short-course radiotherapy versus long-course chemoradiation comparing rates of local recurrence in patients with T3 rectal cancer: Trans-Tasman Radiation Oncology Group trial 01.04. J Clin Oncol 2012;30(31):3827–33. http://dx.doi.org/10.1200/JCO.2012.42.9597 [Erratum in J Clin Oncol 2013 Jan 20;31(3):399].

18. Bujko K, Nowacki MP, Nasierowska-Guttmejer A, et al. Sphincter preservation following preoperative radiotherapy for rectal cancer: report of a randomised trial comparing short-term radiotherapy vs. conventionally fractionated radiochemotherapy. Radiother Oncol 2004;72:15–24.

19. Glimelius B, Påhlman L. Preoperative radiotherapy for rectal cancer: hypofractionation with multiple fractions (15-25 Gy). Ann Ital Chir 2001;72(5):539–47.

20. Frykholm GJ, Isacsson U, Nygård K, et al. Preoperative radiotherapy in rectal carcinoma—aspects of acute adverse effects and radiation technique. Int J Radiat Oncol Biol Phys 1996;35(5):1039–48.

21. Duthoy W, De Gersem W, Vergote K, et al. Clinical implementation of intensity-modulated arc therapy (IMAT) for rectal cancer. Int J Radiat Oncol Biol Phys 2004;60(3):794–806.

22. Jones WE 3rd, Thomas CR Jr, Herman JM, et al. ACR appropriateness criteria® resectable rectal cancer. Radiat Oncol 2012;7:161. http://dx.doi.org/10.1186/1748-717X-7-161.

23. Gevaert T, Engels B, Garibaldi C, et al. Implementation of HybridArc treatment technique in preoperative radiotherapy of rectal cancer: dose patterns in target lesions and organs at risk as compared to helical Tomotherapy and RapidArc. Radiat Oncol 2012;7:120.

24. Mok H, Crane CH, Palmer MB, et al. Intensity modulated radiation therapy (IMRT): differences in target volumes and improvement in clinically relevant doses to small bowel in rectal carcinoma. Radiat Oncol 2011;6:63. http://dx.doi.org/10.1186/1748-717X-6-63.

25. Garofalo M, Moughan J, Hong T, et al. RTOG 0822: a phase II study of preoperative (PREOP) chemoradiotherapy (CRT) utilizing IMRT in combination with capecitabine (C) and oxaliplatin (O) for patients with locally advanced rectal cancer. Int J Radiat Oncol Biol Phys 2011;81(Suppl 2):S3–4.

26. Peeters KC, van de Velde CJ, Leer JW, et al. Late side effects of short-course preoperative radiotherapy combined with total mesorectal excision for rectal cancer: increased bowel dysfunction in irradiated patients-a Dutch Colorectal Cancer Group Study. J Clin Oncol 2005;23(25):6199–206.

27. Marijnen CA, van de Velde CJ, Putter H, et al. Impact of short-term preoperative radiotherapy on health-related quality of life and sexual functioning in primary rectal cancer: report of a multicenter randomized trial. J Clin Oncol 2005; 23(9):1847–58.

28. Gastrointestinal Tumor Study Group. Radiation therapy and fluorouracil with or without semustine for the treatment of patients with surgical adjuvant adenocarcinoma of the rectum. J Clin Oncol 1992;10(4):549–57.

29. Moertel CG, Fleming TR, Macdonald JS, et al. Levamisole and fluorouracil for adjuvant therapy of resected colon cancer. N Engl J Med 1990;322:352–8.

30. Gerard JP, Chapet O, Nemoz C, et al. Preoperative radiotherapy with or without concurrent fluorouracil and leucovorin in T3-4 rectal cancers: results of FFCD 9203. J Clin Oncol 2006;24(28):4620–5. http://dx.doi.org/10.1200/JCO.2006. 06.7629.

31. Bosset JF, Collette L, Calais G, et al. Chemotherapy with preoperative radiotherapy in rectal cancer. N Engl J Med 2006;355:1114–23.

32. De Paoli A, Chiara S, Luppi G, et al. Capecitabine in combination with preoperative radiation therapy in locally advanced, resectable, rectal cancer: a multicentric phase II study. Ann Oncol 2006;17(2):246–51.

33. Hofheinz RD, Wenz F, Post S, et al. Chemoradiotherapy with capecitabine versus fluorouracil for locally advanced rectal cancer: a randomised, multicentre, non-inferiority, phase 3 trial. Lancet Oncol 2012;13(6):579–88. http://dx.doi.org/10.1016/S1470-2045(12)70116-X.

34. Wong SJ, Winter K, Meropol NJ, et al. Radiation Therapy Oncology Group 0247: a randomized Phase II study of neoadjuvant capecitabine and irinotecan or capecitabine and oxaliplatin with concurrent radiotherapy for patients with locally advanced rectal cancer. Int J Radiat Oncol Biol Phys 2012;82(4):1367–75. http://dx.doi.org/10.1016/j.ijrobp.2011.05.027.

35. Gérard JP, Azria D, Gourgou-Bourgade S, et al. Comparison of two neoadjuvant chemoradiotherapy regimens for locally advanced rectal cancer: results of the phase III trial ACCORD 12/0405-Prodige 2. J Clin Oncol 2010;28(10):1638–44.

36. Mohiuddin M, Winter K, Mitchell E, et al. Randomized phase II study of neoadjuvant combined-modality chemoradiation for distal rectal cancer: Radiation Therapy Oncology Group Trial 0012. J Clin Oncol 2006;24(4):650–5.

37. Gollins S, Sun Myint A, Haylock B, et al. Preoperative chemoradiotherapy using concurrent capecitabine and irinotecan in magnetic resonance imaging-defined locally advanced rectal cancer: impact on long-term clinical outcomes. J Clin Oncol 2011;29(8):1042–9. http://dx.doi.org/10.1200/JCO.2010.29.7697.

38. Crane CH, Eng C, Feig BW, et al. Phase II trial of neoadjuvant bevacizumab, capecitabine, and radiotherapy for locally advanced rectal cancer. Int J Radiat Oncol Biol Phys 2010;76(3):824–30. http://dx.doi.org/10.1016/j.ijrobp.2009.02.037.

39. Weiss C, Arnold D, Dellas K, et al. Preoperative radiotherapy of advanced rectal cancer with capecitabine and oxaliplatin with or without cetuximab: a pooled analysis of three prospective phase I-II trials. Int J Radiat Oncol Biol Phys 2010;78(2):472–8. http://dx.doi.org/10.1016/j.ijrobp.2009.07.1718.

40. Glynne-Jones R, Mawdsley S, Harrison M. Cetuximab and chemoradiation for rectal cancer–is the water getting muddy? Acta Oncol 2010;49(3):278–86. http://dx.doi.org/10.3109/02841860903536010.

41. Marijnen CA, Nagtegaal ID, Klein Kranenbarg E, et al, Pathology Review Committee and the Cooperative Clinical Investigators. No downstaging after short-term preoperative radiotherapy in rectal cancer patients. J Clin Oncol 2001; 19:1976–84.

42. Graf W, Dahlberg M, Osman MM, et al. Short-term preoperative radiotherapy results in down-staging of rectal cancer: a study of 1316 patients. Radiother Oncol 1997;43(2):133–7.

43. Latkauskas T, Pauzas H, Gineikiene I, et al. Initial results of a randomized controlled trial comparing clinical and pathological downstaging of rectal cancer after preoperative short-course radiotherapy or long-term chemoradiotherapy, both with delayed surgery. Colorectal Dis 2012;14(3):294–8. http://dx.doi.org/10.1111/j.1463-1318.2011.02815.x.

44. Latkauskas T, Paskauskas S, Dambrauskas Z, et al. Preoperative chemoradiation vs radiation alone for stage II and III resectable rectal cancer: a meta-analysis. Colorectal Dis 2010;12(11):1075–83. http://dx.doi.org/10.1111/j.1463-1318.2009.02015.x.

45. Pettersson D, Cedermark B, Holm T, et al. Interim analysis of the Stockholm III trial of preoperative radiotherapy regimens for rectal cancer. Br J Surg 2010;97(4):580–7. http://dx.doi.org/10.1002/bjs.6914.

46. Rödel C, Martus P, Papadoupolos T, et al. Prognostic significance of tumor regression after preoperative chemoradiotherapy for rectal cancer. J Clin Oncol 2005;23(34):8688–96.

47. Capirci C, Valentini V, Cionini L, et al. Prognostic value of pathologic complete response after neoadjuvant therapy in locally advanced rectal cancer: long-term analysis of 566 ypCR patients. Int J Radiat Oncol Biol Phys 2008;72(1):99–107. http://dx.doi.org/10.1016/j.ijrobp.2007.12.019.

48. Maas M, Nelemans PJ, Valentini V, et al. Long-term outcome in patients with a pathological complete response after chemoradiation for rectal cancer: a pooled analysis of individual patient data. Lancet Oncol 2010;11(9):835–44. http://dx.doi.org/10.1016/S1470-2045(10)70172-8.

49. Habr-Gama A, Perez RO, Nadalin W, et al. Operative versus nonoperative treatment for stage 0 distal rectal cancer following chemoradiation therapy: long-term results. Ann Surg 2004;240(4):711–7 [discussion: 717–8].

50. Habr-Gama A, Perez R, Proscurshim I, et al. Complete clinical response after neoadjuvant chemoradiation for distal rectal cancer. Surg Oncol Clin N Am 2010;19(4):829–45. http://dx.doi.org/10.1016/j.soc.2010.08.001.

51. Smith FM, Chang KH, Sheahan K, et al. The surgical significance of residual mucosal abnormalities in rectal cancer following neoadjuvant chemoradiotherapy. Br J Surg 2012;99(7):993–1001. http://dx.doi.org/10.1002/bjs. 8700.

52. Glynne-Jones R, Hughes R. Critical appraisal of the 'wait and see' approach in rectal cancer for clinical complete responders after chemoradiation. Br J Surg 2012;99(7):897–909. http://dx.doi.org/10.1002/bjs. 8732.

53. Habr-Gama A, Perez RO, Sabbaga J, et al. Increasing the rates of complete response to neoadjuvant chemoradiotherapy for distal rectal cancer: results of a prospective study using additional chemotherapy during the resting period. Dis Colon Rectum 2009;52(12):1927–34. http://dx.doi.org/10.1007/DCR.0b013e3181ba14ed.

54. Rödel C, Arnold D, Becker H, et al. Induction chemotherapy before chemoradiotherapy and surgery for locally advanced rectal cancer: is it time for a randomized phase III trial? Strahlenther Onkol 2010;186(12):658–64. http://dx.doi.org/10.1007/s00066-010-2194-2.

55. NCCN guidelines. Available at: http://www.nccn.org/professionals/physician_gls/pdf/rectal.pdf.

56. NIH/NCI guidelines. Available at: http://www.cancer.gov/cancertopics/pdq/treatment/rectal/HealthProfessional/Page4#Section_43; http://www.cancer.gov/cancertopics/pdq/treatment/rectal/Patient/page4.

57. Peeters KC, Marijnen CA, Nagtegaal ID, et al, Dutch Colorectal Cancer Group. The TME trial after a median follow-up of 6 years: increased local control but no survival benefit in irradiated patients with resectable rectal carcinoma. Ann Surg 2007;246(5):693–701.

58. Sebag-Montefiore D, Stephens RJ, Steele R, et al, on behalf of all the trial collaborators. Preoperative radiotherapy versus selective postoperative chemoradiotherapy in patients with rectal cancer (MRC CR07 and NCIC-CTG C016): a multicentre, randomised trial. Lancet 2009;373(9666):811–20. http://dx.doi.org/10.1016/S0140-6736(09)60484-0.

59. Merchant NB, Guillem JG, Paty PB, et al. T3N0 rectal cancer: results following sharp mesorectal excision and no adjuvant therapy. J Gastrointest Surg 1999; 3(6):642–7.

60. Picon AI, Moore HG, Sternberg SS, et al. Prognostic significance of depth of gross or microscopic perirectal fat invasion in T3 N0 M0 rectal cancers following sharp mesorectal excision and no adjuvant therapy. Int J Colorectal Dis 2003; 18(6):487–92.

61. Willett CG, Badizadegan K, Ancukiewicz M, et al. Prognostic factors in stage T3N0 rectal cancer: do all patients require postoperative pelvic irradiation and chemotherapy? Dis Colon Rectum 1999;42(2):167–73.

62. Gunderson LL, Sargent DJ, Tepper JE, et al. Impact of T and N substage on survival and disease relapse in adjuvant rectal cancer: a pooled analysis. Int J Radiat Oncol Biol Phys 2002;54(2):386–96.

63. Guillem JG, Díaz-González JA, Minsky BD, et al. cT3N0 rectal cancer: potential overtreatment with preoperative chemoradiotherapy is warranted. J Clin Oncol 2008;26(3):368–73. http://dx.doi.org/10.1200/JCO.2007.13.5434.

64. Lombardi R, Cuicchi D, Pinto C, et al. Clinically-staged T3N0 rectal cancer: is preoperative chemoradiotherapy the optimal treatment? Ann Surg Oncol 2010;17(3):838–45. http://dx.doi.org/10.1245/s10434-009-0796-7.

65. Heald RJ, O'Neill BD, Moran B, et al. MRI in predicting curative resection of rectal cancer: new dilemma in multidisciplinary team management. BMJ 2006; 333(7572):808. http://dx.doi.org/10.1136/bmj.333.7572.808.

66. Taylor FG, Quirke P, Heald RJ, et al, MERCURY study group. Preoperative high-resolution magnetic resonance imaging can identify good prognosis stage I, II, and III rectal cancer best managed by surgery alone: a prospective, multicenter, European study. Ann Surg 2011;253(4):711–9. http://dx.doi.org/10.1097/SLA.0b013e31820b8d52.

67. Benson R, Wong CS, Cummings BJ, et al. Local excision and postoperative radiotherapy for distal rectal cancer. Int J Radiat Oncol Biol Phys 2001;50(5): 1309–16. http://dx.doi.org/10.1016/S0360-3016(01)01545-0.

68. Chakravarti A, Compton CC, Shellito PC, et al. Long-term follow-up of patients with rectal cancer managed by local excision with and without adjuvant irradiation. Ann Surg 1999;230(1):49–54. http://dx.doi.org/10.1097/00000658-199907000-00008.

69. Mendenhall WM, Morris CG, Rout WR, et al. Local excision and postoperative radiation therapy for rectal adenocarcinoma. Int J Cancer 2001;(Suppl 96): 89–96.

70. Greenberg JA, Shibata D, Herndon JE 2nd, et al. Local excision of distal rectal cancer: an update of cancer and leukemia group B 8984. Dis Colon Rectum 2008;51(8):1185–91. http://dx.doi.org/10.1007/s10350-008-9231-6 [discussion: 1191–4].

71. Borschitz T, Wachtlin D, Möhler M, et al. Neoadjuvant chemoradiation and local excision for T2-3 rectal cancer. Ann Surg Oncol 2008;15(3):712–20.

72. Bonnen M, Crane C, Vauthey JN, et al. Long-term results using local excision after preoperative chemoradiation among selected T3 rectal cancer patients. Int J Radiat Oncol Biol Phys 2004;60(4):1098–105.

73. Belluco C, De Paoli A, Canzonieri V, et al. Long-term outcome of patients with complete pathologic response after neoadjuvant chemoradiation for cT3 rectal cancer: implications for local excision surgical strategies. Ann Surg Oncol 2011; 18(13):3686–93. http://dx.doi.org/10.1245/s10434-011-1822-0.

74. Marks JH, Valsdottir EB, DeNittis A, et al. Transanal endoscopic microsurgery for the treatment of rectal cancer: comparison of wound complication rates with and without neoadjuvant radiation therapy. Surg Endosc 2009;23(5): 1081–7. http://dx.doi.org/10.1007/s00464-009-0326-5.

75. Perez RO, Habr-Gama A, São Julião GP, et al. Transanal endoscopic microsurgery for residual rectal cancer after neoadjuvant chemoradiation therapy is associated with significant immediate pain and hospital readmission rates. Dis Colon Rectum 2011;54(5):545–51. http://dx.doi.org/10.1007/DCR.0b013e3182083b84.

76. Callender GG, Das P, Rodriguez-Bigas MA, et al. Local excision after preoperative chemoradiation results in an equivalent outcome to total mesorectal excision in selected patients with T3 rectal cancer. Ann Surg Oncol 2010;17(2): 441–7. http://dx.doi.org/10.1245/s10434-009-0735-7.

77. Bökkerink GM, de Graaf EJ, Punt CJ, et al. The CARTS study: chemoradiation therapy for rectal cancer in the distal rectum followed by organ-sparing transanal endoscopic microsurgery. BMC Surg 2011;11:34. http://dx.doi.org/10.1186/1471-2482-11-34.

78. Mendenhall WM, Rout WR, Vauthey JN, et al. Conservative treatment of rectal adenocarcinoma with endocavitary irradiation or wide local excision and postoperative irradiation. J Clin Oncol 1997;15(10):3241–8.

79. Coatmeur O, Truc G, Barillot I, et al. Treatment of T1-T2 rectal tumors by contact therapy and interstitial brachytherapy. Radiother Oncol 2004;70(2):177–82.

80. Christoforidis D, McNally MP, Jarosek SL, et al. Endocavitary contact radiation therapy for ultrasonographically staged T1 N0 and T2 N0 rectal cancer. Br J Surg 2009;96(4):430–6. http://dx.doi.org/10.1002/bjs.6478.

81. Lavertu S, Schild SE, Gunderson LL, et al. Endocavitary radiation therapy for rectal adenocarcinoma: 10-year results. Am J Clin Oncol 2003;26(5):508–12.

82. Aumock A, Birnbaum EH, Fleshman JW, et al. Treatment of rectal adenocarcinoma with endocavitary and external beam radiotherapy: results for 199 patients with localized tumors. Int J Radiat Oncol Biol Phys 2001;51(2):363–70.

83. Winslow ER, Kodner IJ, Mutch MG, et al. Outcome of salvage abdominoperineal resection after failed endocavitary radiation in patients with rectal cancer. Dis Colon Rectum 2004;47(12):2039–46.

84. Hesselager C, Vuong T, Påhlman L, et al. Neoadjuvant high dose endorectal brachytherapy or short course external beam radiotherapy in resectable rectal cancer. Colorectal Dis 2013. http://dx.doi.org/10.1111/codi.12193.

85. Vuong T, Devic S, Podgorsak E. High dose rate endorectal brachytherapy as a neoadjuvant treatment for patients with resectable rectal cancer. Clin Oncol (R Coll Radiol) 2007;19(9):701–5.

Controversies in Abdominoperineal Excision

Torbjörn Holm, MD, PhD

KEYWORDS

- Rectal cancer • Abdominoperineal excision • Circumferential resection margin
- Intraoperative bowel perforation • Local recurrence • Cancer survival
- Perineal reconstruction

KEY POINTS

- Oncological outcomes after abdominoperineal excision (APE) in rectal cancer have not improved to the same extent as those seen after AR.
- The conventional synchronous combined APE is not a standardized procedure.
- Depending on tumor stage and patient characteristics and based on well-defined anatomic structures, three types of APE can be described, which differ in the extent of removed tissue.
- A more precise surgical approach may reduce tumor-involved resection margins and intraoperative bowel perforations, which likely will improve local control and survival for patients with low rectal cancer.

INTRODUCTION

The earliest surgical attempts to treat rectal cancer were via the perineum and the techniques used were exclusively extraperitoneal with extremely poor results. The perioperative mortality was high, functional results appalling, and local control very bad, with local recurrence rates up to 90%. Sir Ernest Miles, a surgeon at St Mark's Hospital in London, took an important step in the development of surgery for rectal cancer when he published an article, "A Method of Performing Abdomino-Perineal Excision for Carcinoma of the Rectum and of the Terminal Portion of the Pelvic Colon," on December 19, 1908, in *The Lancet*.[1] This was a thorough description of an APE of the rectum and has since been called the *Miles operation*. In his original description of the procedure, the rectum was bluntly mobilized down to the sacrococcygeal articulation, to the prostate, and to "the upper surface of the levatores ani" laterally, thus leaving the mesorectum attached to the pelvic floor. After this mobilization of the

No disclosures.

Section of Coloproctology, Department of Surgical Gastroenterology, Karolinska University Hospital, Stockholm 171 76, Sweden

E-mail address: torbjorn.holm@karolinska.se

Surg Oncol Clin N Am 23 (2014) 93–111

http://dx.doi.org/10.1016/j.soc.2013.09.005

1055-3207/14/$ – see front matter © 2014 Elsevier Inc. All rights reserved.

surgonc.theclinics.com

rectum, a colostomy was created and the abdominal wall was closed. The patient was turned over and placed in the right lateral and semiprone position. Miles emphasized that the levator muscles should be divided "as far outwards as their origin from the white line so as to include the lateral zone of spread"; therefore, the perineal part of the operation included a wide excision of skin, fat, and pelvic floor (levator muscles).

The Lancet article had an enormous impact on the surgical community and for many decades the Miles operation was the gold standard procedure for all rectal carcinomas. The concept of removing the entire rectum, the anus, and the perineum in all patients with rectal cancer, however, was gradually abandoned. Increasing experience with bowel reconstruction, including developments of stapling instruments, led to a new concept of anterior resection (AR) and low AR (LAR), which became the standard procedures for tumors of the upper and middle rectum.[2–6]

For tumors of the lower rectum, most surgeons continued to perform APE, although the extensive perineal approach described by Miles was more or less neglected and the synchronous combined APE was introduced as a feasible procedure that became popular and gained widespread use in the treatment of low rectal cancer.[7] During the synchronous combined operation, the perineal part is carried out simultaneously with the pelvic part of the abdominal procedure, with the patient in the supine lithotomy, or Lloyd-Davies position; the rectum with its mesorectum is first mobilized down to the pelvic floor and the perineal surgeon then enters the pelvic cavity just in front of the coccyx, the levator muscles are divided on both sides, and, finally, the rectum is dissected off the prostate or the vagina and the specimen is delivered through the perineum.

Although there were gradual improvements in the treatment of rectal cancer during the twentieth century, local control remained a major problem after surgery, with local recurrence rates of up to 40% after potentially curative resections.[8] Therefore, irradiation to the rectum and to the pelvis, both preoperatively and postoperatively, was tried in order to improve local control. Preoperative radiotherapy has been evaluated in several large randomized trials and was shown to reduce local recurrence rates by 50% and to improve cancer-specific survival.[9,10]

With the development of total mesorectal excision (TME), as described by Heald and colleagues,[11,12] treatment results improved dramatically, both concerning local control and survival. Heald and colleagues[11] reported a local recurrence rate of approximately 5% and a cancer-specific survival of approximately 70% at 5 years, without radiotherapy.[12] Initially, these results were mistrusted by many surgeons but, due to extensive educational efforts, the technique was gradually accepted.[13] During the recent 15 to 20 years, the TME technique for rectal cancer resection has been introduced in many countries and, subsequently, the results with regard to local control and cancer survival have improved significantly. Local recurrence rates are now reported to be less than 10% in population-based studies.[14,15] The acknowledgment of TME as the standard surgical technique in the treatment of rectal cancer has resulted not only in improved local control and survival but also in increasing rates of sphincter-saving procedures and improved results concerning urogenital function.

Consequently, in the past 15 to 20 years, teaching rectal cancer surgery mainly focused on the operative technique of TME and AR. Although the technique used for the abdominal part of an APE was modified along the lines of TME, little attention was given to the perineal part of this procedure. Thus, most surgeons adopted the technique of sharp dissection under direct vision outside the mesorectal fascia down to the pelvic floor, with the aim of saving autonomic nerves and creating perfect specimen with an intact mesorectal fascia. The perineal part, however, was often completed in the conventional way, with dissection close to the external sphincter and with the division of the levator muscles close to the rectal wall. With a patient in the supine lithotomy position, it is difficult to achieve an optimal view, especially anteriorly, and, therefore, parts of the perineal dissection are often done with blunt dissection when this approach is used.

PROBLEMS RELATED TO THE CONVENTIONAL SYNCHRONOUS COMBINED APE

In recent years, several investigators have acknowledged that local control and survival after APE have not improved to the same degree as those seen after AR. In one study based on 561 patients from Leeds, United Kingdom, it was reported that patients undergoing APE had a higher local failure rate (22.3% vs 13.5%) and a poorer survival (52.3% vs 65.8%) compared with patients who had an AR during the same time period.[16]

Another article based on data from five different European trials reported that the APE procedure was associated with an increased risk of circumferential resection margin (CRM) involvement, an increased local recurrence rate, and a decreased cancer-specific survival.[17] A large cohort study from Norway also reported a higher local recurrence rate (15% vs 10%) and a poorer 5-year survival (55% vs 68%) after APE than after AR.[15]

These differences in oncological outcomes between the two procedures may be explained by several factors, including anatomic difficulties and the surgical technique associated with standard APE surgery. In the lower rectum, the surrounding mesorectum is reduced in size and disappears at the top of the sphincters. Below this level, the sphincter muscle forms the CRM. As discussed previously, the abdominal dissection during a conventional synchronous combined APE is often carried out along the mesorectum, all the way down to the pelvic floor and the top of the puborectalis muscle, with the mesorectum mobilized off the levator muscles. The perineal dissection then follows the external sphincter to meet the pelvic dissection at the top of the anal canal (**Fig. 1**A). With this technique the retrieved specimen often has a typical waist at 3 to 5 cm from the distal end, corresponding to the top of the external sphincter at the level of the puborectalis muscle and the lowest part of the mesorectum (see **Fig. 1**B).

This inward coning at the pelvic floor carries the dissection close to the rectal wall and several studies have reported higher rates of bowel perforation and tumor involvement of CRM after APE compared with AR. Nagtegaal and colleagues[18] assessed 846 AR specimens and 373 APE specimens from the Dutch TME trial and found that the plane of resection was within the sphincter muscle, the submucosa, or lumen in more than one-third of the APE cases, and in the remainder was on the sphincter muscles. This resulted in a positive CRM rate of 30.4% after APE versus 10.7% after AR and a perforation rate of 13.7% after APE versus 2.5% after AR. Similarly, population-based reports from Sweden, Norway, and Holland have shown a 3-fold increase in perforation rates after APE compared with AR (14%–15% vs 3%–4%) and that perforation is a significant risk factor for adverse outcomes regarding local control and survival.[19] In addition, a publication based on the Dutch TME trial reported that tumor involvement of the CRM was an independent risk factor, both for local recurrence and survival, in patients undergoing APE.[20] Thus, the differences in oncological outcomes between the conventional type of APE and AR may to a substantial part be explained by the increased risk of tumor-involved margins and inadvertent bowel perforations, because both these factors are significantly related to local control and survival.

With the development of TME leading to substantially improved results after AR, many surgeons have advocated low or ultralow AR, even for tumors of the lower

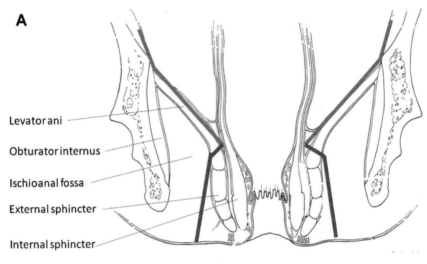

Levator ani

Obturator internus

Ischioanal fossa

External sphincter

Internal sphincter

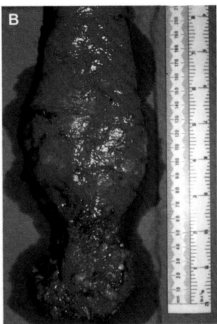

Fig. 1. (*A*) The pelvic dissection in a conventional synchronous combined APE is carried along outside the mesorectal fascia down to the top of the anal canal (*blue line*) and the perineal dissection is carried along the external sphincter (*red line*). The two dissection planes meet at the level of the puborectal muscle, which creates a waist on the specimen. (*B*) Photograph of a fresh specimen after a conventional APE, with the typical waist at the level of the puborectal muscle.

rectum. It has also been shown that these procedures are feasible and oncologically safe, provided that the tumor can be removed with a clear distal and circumferential margin. In dedicated and highly specialized centers, adopting intersphincteric AR for appropriate cases, the overall APE rate may be below 10%.

The functional results after an ultralow AR may be poor, however, especially if patients have received preoperative radiochemotherapy.[21] In patients with a preoperative history of gas or fecal incontinence, careful counseling is, therefore, mandatory and information should be given about the risk of a poor functional outcome after AR. In such patients, a permanent stoma may be preferable.

If a tumor in the lower rectum is more advanced, growing close to or into the distal mesorectal fascia, the levator muscle, or the external sphincter and, thereby, threatens the potential CRM, it may not be possible to perform a safe AR and in these cases an APE is necessary. The decision of when to recommend an APE is, therefore, related to both the patient and the tumor characteristics. Because such variables are interpreted differently between different surgeons, the rate of APE varies greatly between individual surgeons and between different institutions. Morris and colleagues[22] reported that the rate of APE varied from 8.5% to 52.6% between different English hospitals. In Sweden, the rate of APE for low rectal cancer, as defined by tumors within 6 cm from the anal verge, has varied between 80% and 92% during the past 15 years (**Fig. 2**). Thus, APE is still a common operation for low rectal cancer and because the results have been suboptimal, it is important to change the concept of APE in order to reduce the rate of inadvertent bowel perforations and tumor-involved margins and, thereby, obtain improved oncological outcomes.

THE NEW CONCEPT OF APE

One problem associated with the conventional type of synchronous combined APE is the lack of standardization and a clear definition of the details of the perineal part of this procedure.[23] Although the abdominal part of the operation follows the standard TME principles, there has been no agreement on the surgical details of the perineal part of the operation. This probably explains the significant variability in the observed rates of tumor-involved margins, bowel perforations, local recurrence, and survival.[24] Due to this variability and the suboptimal results after APE, there has been a call for a different concept and a more standardized approach to APE.[25] In recent years, a new concept of APE has, therefore, evolved, which takes into account the specific anatomic structures of the perineum and the pelvic floor and which aims to adopt and standardize the procedure according to the characteristics of the patient and the tumor. Basically, three types of APE can be described in relation to the perineal

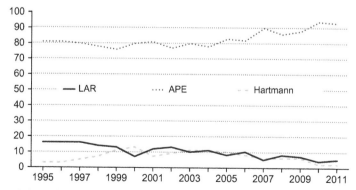

Fig. 2. Graph from the Swedish Rectal Cancer Registry showing the proportion of patients with rectal cancer below 6 cm, operated on with APE, LAR, or Hartmann procedure annually since 1995. (*Adapted from* Påhlman L, Bohe M, Cedermark B, et al. The Swedish rectal cancer registry. Br J Surg 2007;94(10):1285–92; with permission.)

approach and the extent of dissection—the intersphincteric APE, the extralavator APE (ELAPE), and the ischioanal APE—and the indications are different for these three procedures (shown in **Box 1**).

Surgical Considerations

A preoperative local and distant staging is fundamental in the management of patients with rectal cancer. The objective is to assess the local extent of the tumor and to detect distant metastases. The local staging of rectal cancer is especially important in low tumors because the extent of the procedure is related to the height and the size of the cancer and the depth of infiltration into the rectal wall and surrounding structures (T stage). High-resolution MRI has evolved as the tool of choice for local staging in rectal cancer, sometimes followed by ultrasonography to distinguish between early tumors (T1–T2). CT of the chest, abdomen, and pelvis is the preferred modality for distant staging and should be performed in all patients.

As for all surgical operations, patients planned for an APE should be well informed about the extent of the procedure, the potential complications that may occur postoperatively, and the possible late sequellae, such as urogenital dysfunction and stoma problems. A crucial part of the preoperative preparation is to have patients meet a stoma nurse well ahead of the operation. The stoma nurse has an important role in informing the patient about the practicalities of stoma care and appliances. It is also important that the placement of the stoma is carefully assessed to avoid a suboptimal placement, close to a skin fold or a scar. Patients need to be able to see the stoma and this may be a problem in obese patients if the stoma is placed too low. Thus, the stoma site should always be marked in advance by a stoma nurse.

The preoperative preparation should also always include prophylaxis against postoperative deep venous thromboembolism and postoperative infections but per oral mechanical bowel preparation is not necessary for APE.

For all three types of APE, the abdominal part of the operation is the same and includes the mobilization of the left colon and the rectum down to the top of the levator muscles, ligation and division of the inferior mesenteric artery or superior rectal artery, ligation and division of the inferior mesenteric vein, and division of the colon, usually at the level between the descending and the sigmoid colon.

Box 1
Indications for APE in rectal cancer

Intersphincteric APE

- Patient unsuitable for bowel reconstruction
- Preoperative history of incontinence
- High risk of anastomotic leak
- Comorbidity: crucial to prevent leakage + fatal outcome
- Patient preference

ELAPE

- Tumor extending less than 1 cm from dentate line (T2–T4 cancer)
- Tumor threatening CRM

Ischioanal APE

- Locally advanced cancer infiltrating levator muscles, ischioanal fat, or perianal skin
- Perforated cancer with abscess or fistula in ischioanal compartment

The mobilization of the rectum and the mesorectum during the pelvic dissection in the abdominal part of the operation differs, however, between the intersphincteric APE and the two other types, and the perineal dissection is different for the three different types of APE (described later). The abdominal part of an APE, including the pelvic dissection, can be done either open, with laparotomy, or with minimally invasive techniques.

INTERSPHINCTERIC APE

An intersphincteric APE is indicated when a low anastomosis is undesirable for different reasons, for example, in patients with a preoperative history of incontinence or with a high risk of anastomotic leakage. It may also be an option in patients who have had a previous AR and who need to have their neorectum and anastomosis removed due to anastomotic leakage and chronic pelvic sepsis. The pelvic dissection in intersphincteric APE is identical to that performed for AR, which includes the mobilization of the rectum with an intact mesorectum down to the pelvic floor and the puborectalis muscle. Because an intersphincteric APE is not performed when the tumor is close to the anus, a transverse stapler can be put across the rectum, just above the puborectal sling, to seal the bowel and to prevent leakage of mucus or feces from the anus during the perineal part of this procedure.

The Perineal Part of the Intersphincteric APE

Once the rectum and mesorectum has been mobilized down to the top of the anal canal, the patient's legs are elevated and the perineum exposed. The surgeon and assistant now move from the abdomen to perform the perineal phase of the intersphincteric APE. The anal canal is washed out and an incision is made around the anus just distal to the intersphincteric groove. A self-retaining retractor with hooks is recommended to optimize the view and to facilitate the intersphincteric dissection. Once the skin incision is made, the anus is closed with a running suture. The dissection then follows the intersphincteric plane between the internal and external sphincter, around the circumference of the anal canal, and all the way up to the puborectal sling and into the pelvic cavity (**Fig. 3**A). The specimen is then gently removed either through the perineal incision or, if the mesorectum is large and bulky, lifted up from the pelvis and removed from the abdomen via the abdominal incision (see **Fig. 3**B).

The perineal incision is then closed with a running or interrupted suture in the puborectalis and external sphincter. It is the author's preference to use a running suture in three layers, where the most superficial suture line is placed subdermal to leave the skin unsealed in order to allow for discharge of fluid from the wound.

EXTRALEVATOR APE

ELAPE is indicated in patients with tumors threatening the external sphincter or levator muscle and where an ultralow AR or an intersphincteric APE would not achieve a clear CRM (**Fig. 4**). The main purpose is thus to reduce the risk of inadvertent bowel perforation and CRM involvement. As described later, this can be accomplished because the levator muscles are excised en bloc with the mesorectum, to protect the most distal part of the bowel, thereby avoiding the waist of the specimen, which has been so common after the conventional type of synchronous combined APE. Because the levator muscles should not be separated from the mesorectum, the pelvic dissection during the abdominal part of an ELAPE differs notably from an AR or an intersphincteric APE.

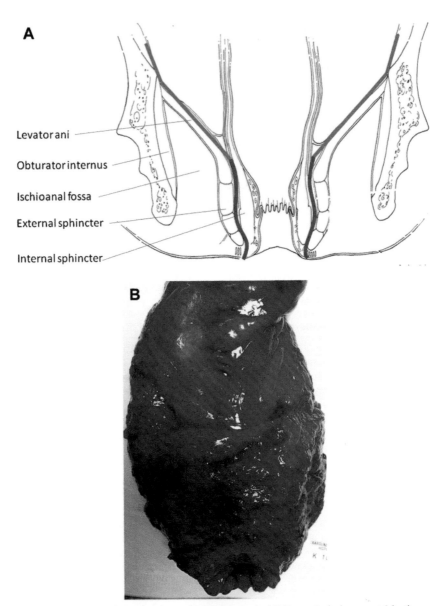

Levator ani

Obturator internus

Ischioanal fossa

External sphincter

Internal sphincter

Fig. 3. (*A*) The pelvic dissection in an intersphincteric APE is carried along outside the mesorectal fascia down to the top of the anal canal (*blue line*) and the perineal dissection is carried out between the internal and external anal sphincter (*red line*). The two dissection planes meet at the level of the puborectal muscle. (*B*) Photograph showing a fresh specimen after an intersphincteric APE.

The Pelvic Dissection in ELAPE

The initial abdominal and pelvic dissection is identical to that described previously but with one important difference. In both AR and intersphincteric APE, the dissection continues all the way down to the pelvic floor and the puborectalis muscle and

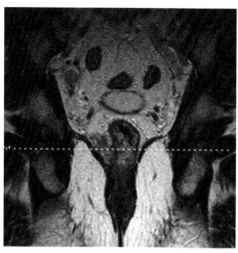

Fig. 4. MRI showing a low rectal cancer threatening the levator muscle.

subsequently the mesorectum is lifted off the levator muscles. In ELAPE, it is crucial not to take the mobilization of the rectum and mesorectum as far down as the pelvic floor. Instead, the dissection should proceed only down to the sacrococcygeal junction dorsally, just beyond the inferior hypogastric plexus anterolaterally, and anteriorly dissection should stop just below the seminal vesicles in men or the cervix uteri in women. By terminating the mobilization of the rectum and mesorectum at this level, the mesorectum is still attached to the levator muscles of the pelvic floor, which is a crucial feature of the ELAPE (**Fig. 5A**).

The Perineal Part of the ELAPE

The perineal part of the ELAPE differs considerably from the perineal part of the intersphincteric APE. This part of the operation can be performed with the patient either in the supine, Lloyd-Davies position, or in the prone, jackknife position. The prone position is often preferable due to the excellent exposure of the operative field. Some surgeons prefer the supine position, mainly to avoid the time-consuming process of turning a patient with subsequent preparation and dressing of the perineal area.

Irrespective of the position, the perineal phase starts with closure of the anus to avoid any spillage of feces or mucus, which may contain tumor cells. In the ELAPE, less skin and ischioanal fat is excised compared with Miles' original description of the APE procedure. After incision of the skin, the external sphincter is identified and the dissection is continued outside the sphincter up to the levator muscles on both sides. The levator muscles are then followed-up to the pelvic sidewall (obturator internus muscle).

Once the external sphincter and levator muscles are exposed around the circumference, the pelvis is entered, either just anterior to the tip of the coccyx or through the sacrococcygeal junction. At this stage, it is important to identify the mesorectum in order not to injure the mesorectal fascia. The pelvic floor (ie, the levator muscle) is now divided and the division continues onto the prostate or vagina. The specimen is still attached to the anterior aspect of the levator muscles and to the prostate or posterior wall of the vagina.

The dissection in the anterior plane during the perineal phase of the ELAPE is the most difficult, and potentially most dangerous, part of the procedure because of the

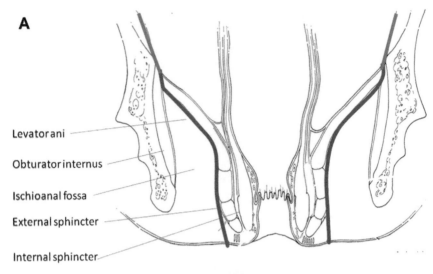

Levator ani
Obturator internus
Ischioanal fossa
External sphincter
Internal sphincter

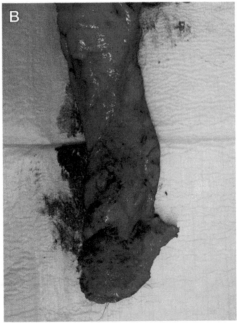

Fig. 5. (*A*) The pelvic dissection in an ELAPE is carried along outside the mesorectal fascia but stops at the top of the levator muscle (*blue line*). The perineal dissection proceeds just outside the external sphincter and along the levator muscle fascia, up to its origin at the obturator internus muscle (*red line*). (*B*) Photograph showing a fresh specimen after an ELAPE. The specimen is more cylindrical, without a waist, because the levator muscle is attached to the mesorectum.

close relationship between the anterior rectal wall and the prostate or posterior vaginal wall. In addition, the neurovascular bundles derived from the inferior hypogastric plexus run anterolaterally on each side of the prostate or vagina and close to the rectum and can easily be damaged if they are not recognized at this stage of the operation (**Fig. 6**). The dissection along the anterior and lateral aspects of the lower rectum must, therefore, be performed meticulously and with great care. If the dissection is performed close to the rectal wall, there is a risk of inadvertent perforation or tumor-involved margin and if the dissection is carried out too laterally, or too anteriorly, there is a risk of damage to the neurovascular bundles or to the prostate or vagina. In anteriorly located tumors, it may be necessary to include the posterior vaginal wall or a slice of the posterior prostate with the specimen and sometimes even to sacrifice the neurovascular bundle on one side, to be able to achieve a negative CRM. This extension of the procedure should, however, ideally be planned in advance, based on the preoperative MRI staging and digital examination, so that the surgeon is prepared for it and so that the patient is well informed about the consequences, which may be impairment of bladder and/or sexual function.

When the perineal dissection is carried out as described, the excised specimen is cylindrical, usually without a waist, because the levator muscle is still attached to the mesorectum, forming a cuff around the rectal muscle tube (see **Fig. 5B**).

THE ISCHIOANAL APE

In some patients, the rectal tumor is locally advanced and may have infiltrated or even perforated the pelvic floor (ie, the levator muscle) (**Fig. 7**). In other patients, a perianal abscess may sometimes be the presenting feature of a perforated low rectal cancer and, after drainage, a fistula may persist between the lower rectum and the perianal skin. In a few very low tumors, the growth may extend into the perianal skin (**Fig. 8**). In these instances, an ELAPE may not be sufficient to achieve a safe, tumor-free CRM and ischioanal APE is usually required to obtain an oncologically secure margin. In this situation, the levator muscle must be removed and covered with ischioanal fat, and the ischioanal fat must be removed to include the perianal fistula, which may

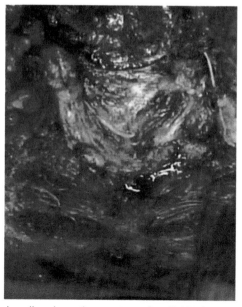

Fig. 6. Neurovascular bundles along the prostate after ELAPE (patient in prone position).

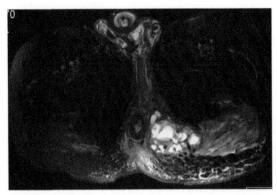

Fig. 7. MRI of a perforated low rectal cancer, penetrating through the levator muscle into the ischioanal space.

contain tumor cells. Therefore, the ischioanal APE is a valid procedure in these special situations.

The abdominal part of the ischioanal APE is exactly equivalent to the abdominal part of the ELAPE. Thus, the dissection stops just above the levator muscle and leaves the mesorectum attached to the pelvic floor (**Fig. 9A**). When the abdominal part of the procedure is completed, with closure of the abdominal wall and formation of a colostomy, the patient is turned into the prone jackknife position.

The Perineal Part of the Ischioanal APE

After proper preparation of the skin of the perineum, lower sacrum, the medial parts of the buttocks, and the vagina in women, a double purse-string suture is placed to close the anus. The area of the skin incision in an ischioanal APE depends on the extent of tumor involvement of the skin. Any tumor infiltration or fistula opening must be included in the excised skin area with a margin of at least 2 to 3 cm. As soon as the

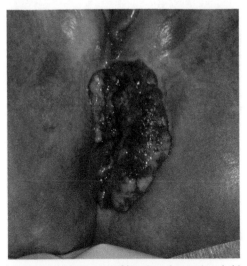

Fig. 8. Low locally advanced rectal cancer infiltrating the perianal skin.

A

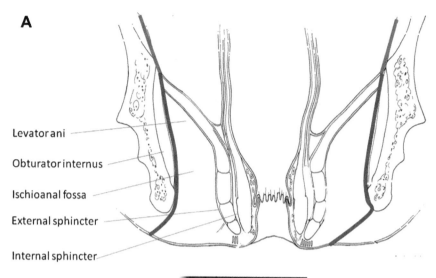

Levator ani

Obturator internus

Ischioanal fossa

External sphincter

Internal sphincter

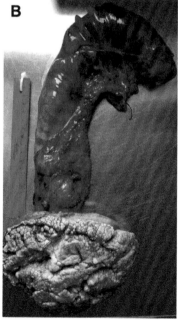

Fig. 9. (*A*) The pelvic dissection in an ischioanal APE is carried along outside the mesorectal fascia but stops at the top of the levator muscle (*blue line*). The perineal dissection is directed toward the ischial tuberosities and follows the obturator internus muscle fascia in order to remove the fat in the ischioanal compartment en bloc (*red line*). The size of the skin incision depends on the extent of tumor involvement in the skin and may be extensive (*left side*) or similar to the skin incision in an ELAPE (*right side*). (*B*) Photograph showing a fresh specimen after an ischioanal APE. In very advanced tumors infiltrating the perineal skin, a wide skin excision and a complete clearance of both ischioanal compartments may be necessary for a potentially curative operation.

incision deepens into the subcutaneous space, the dissection should be directed laterally toward the ischial tuberosity and progresses onto the fascia of the internal obturator muscle. Thus, contrary to an ELAPE, the dissection does not follow the external sphincter and levator muscle but is instead carried along the fascia of the internal obturator muscle. The dissection is performed along this plane up to where the levator muscle is inserted onto the internal obturator muscle and hence includes the entire fat compartment of the ischioanal space. This dissection can be performed unilaterally or bilaterally depending on the extent of tumor growth. When the dissection up to this level is completed, the sacrococcygeal junction is incised and the pelvic cavity is entered in the same fashion as with an ELAPE. The subsequent dissection is also similar to that of the ELAPE, as the levator muscles are divided along the fascia of the internal obturator muscle onto the prostate in men or the vagina in women. Also, the anterior and lateral dissection along the prostate or vagina is carried out as in an ELAPE. As discussed previously, the difference between ELAPE and ischioanal APE is that the fat in the ischioanal space is resected en bloc and attached to the levator muscle (see **Fig. 9**B). This procedure is similar to what Miles described in 1908 in his original article in *The Lancet*.

WHAT ARE THE CURRENT CONTROVERSIES IN APE?

Due to the suboptimal oncological outcomes associated with the conventional type of APE, as reported from individual institutions and from population-based studies, there has recently been an increasing interest in the management of patients with low rectal cancer and calls for a change in approach to APE surgery.[18] The new concept of APE and ELAPE has created a novel interest in the anatomy of the pelvis, and pelvic floor and anatomic cadaver studies and studies on the surgical anatomy of these structures have been published.[26,27] There has also been focus on the local staging of low rectal cancer with MRI and a more accurate radiologic description of the lower rectum, sphincters, and pelvic floor has been suggested.[28]

A description of the extended abdominoperineal resection (or ELAPE) was published in 2007 and since then, increasing numbers of surgeons have used the technique.[29] In 2010, West and colleagues[30] published a comparative study on 176 ELAPE procedures from 11 European colorectal surgeons with 124 standard excisions from one UK center and found that ELAPE removed more tissue from outside the smooth muscle layer and was associated with less CRM involvement and intraoperative perforations (IOPs) than standard surgery. Stelzner and colleagues[31] performed a literature search to identify articles reporting on APE after the introduction of TME and compared outcomes in 1097 patients after ELAPE with 4147 patients after conventional APE. They found significant risk reductions in the rates of inadvertent bowel perforation (4.1% vs 10.4%), CRM involvement (9.6% vs 15.4%), and the rate of local recurrence (6.6% vs 11.9%) and concluded, "extended techniques of APE result in superior oncologic outcome as compared to standard techniques."

Despite seemingly encouraging results after ELAPE, there have been disputes on the necessity of changing from the conventional type of synchronous combined APE to a more extensive procedure. There have been three main issues of disagreement: the extent of perineal dissection and removal of the pelvic floor, the positioning of the patient, and the methods of reconstructing the pelvic floor.

Extent of Perineal Dissection and Removal of the Pelvic Floor

A study from Gothenburg, Sweden, included 158 consecutive patients with rectal cancer undergoing APE between 2004 and 2009; ELAPE was performed in 79 patients and standard APE in 79. There was no significant difference in CRM involvement, rate of IOPs, or local recurrence rate between the groups but the rate of perineal wound complications was higher and hospital stay longer in patients having had an ELAPE. The investigators concluded that their results did not show any advantage for ELAPE.[32]

In 2012, the Mayo group reported results from 655 consecutive patients with rectal cancer treated with curative intent, using surgery alone. All 246 patients having an APE were operated in the Lloyd-Davies position. The local recurrence rate at 5 years was 5.5% and not significantly different from the local recurrence rate after AR. Also, disease-free survival was similar after APE and AR. It was concluded, "commitment to a standardized wide resection should be the current approach to APR."[33] When this article is read in more detail, however, the operative technique for APE is described as follows: "the widest part of the perineal dissection was carried to the ischial tuberosities bilaterally and then extended upwards to incorporate a majority of the pelvic floor, joining the anterior dissection from the pelvic side without coning in." Thus, it is clear that the authors' standard approach to APE is ELAPE, performed in the supine position.

Recently, a review presented by Krishna and colleagues[34] compared outcomes after ELAPE and standard APE and found no significant differences in CRM involvement or IOP and concluded that the role of ELAPE of the rectum should be investigated further in randomized controlled trials.

The problem in comparing ELAPE with standard APE and conventional APE is the lack of definition of the latter two. With the new concept of APE, including ELAPE, there is a clear definition of the planes of dissection and the relevant anatomic landmarks. This has not been the case with conventional, synchronous combined APE and the surgical technique has probably varied considerably, which likely explains the significant differences in local control and survival. It is important to realize that the external sphincter is integrally related to the levator muscle and, therefore, removal of the external sphincter is, by definition, the initial part of an ELAPE. All that really is at issue is thus the extent of levator removal, which has often not been clarified in reports on results after conventional APE. Therefore, it is futile to compare ELAPE with conventional APE unless the exact extent of levator removal has been defined in the latter. When this is done, it may be evident that standard APE is in fact ELAPE, as in the article from the Mayo Clinic.[33]

Positioning of the Patient for APE

In Miles' original description of the APE procedure, the perineal part of the operation was performed in the right lateral and semiprone position after completion of the abdominal phase and the stoma creation. Subsequently, the synchronous combined APE gained popularity and became standard for the vast majority of surgeons. With the conventional synchronous combined APE, the perineal part of the operation was performed with the patient in the supine Lloyd-Davies position and, as described previously, the excised specimen invariably had a waist just proximal to the puborectal sling and often also an inadvertent perforation or an involved CRM.

Due to the increasing awareness of the problems associated with the synchronous combined APE, the ELAPE was introduced as a different and more radical procedure, performed via the posterior perineal approach in the prone jackknife position, which closely mirrors the original Miles operation.[29] The main purpose of the prone jackknife position is to optimize the visibility of the operative field and to have full control of the perineal and pelvic floor anatomy. As a result, the correct anatomic planes can be followed more easily and the risk of perforation or tumor-involved margins can be reduced.

The prone jackknife position during the perineal part of an APE has also been questioned, however, by different investigators. In a study by de Campos-Lobato and colleagues,[35] APE performed in 81 patients in the prone position was compared with the same operation performed in 87 patients in the supine position. No difference was found in local or distant recurrence or survival and the investigators conclude, "surgical positioning during the perineal part of the abdominoperineal resection does not affect perioperative morbidity or oncologic outcomes." Again, from their description, "The levator muscles were entirely dissected off their attachments to the pelvic sidewalls"; it is clear that ELAPE was performed in both the supine and prone positions.

Martijnse and colleagues[36] recently reported that focus on the perineal dissection and a standardized approach in the supine position can reduce CRM involvement substantially.

Thus, it is essential not to confuse positioning with surgical technique, and ELAPE can be applied regardless of whether a patient is placed supine, prone, or in a lateral position. The position is not crucial per se, provided that skilled and properly trained surgeons perform a meticulous dissection to create a perfect specimen in the extralevator plane. Many surgeons prefer the prone position, however, due to better exposure and because it also facilitates teaching.

Reconstruction of the Pelvic Floor

Primary closure of the perineal wound has been the most common method of perineal reconstruction after a synchronous combined APE. Although the clinical course after primary closure is often uneventful, complications due to the perineal wound is one of the major problems associated with the conventional type of APE, especially in patients who have received neoadjuvant treatment. Wound problems, including dehiscence and delayed wound healing, have been reported in up to 50% of patients receiving preoperative radiotherapy after APE with primary wound closure.[37] It may be that these problems become even more frequent in patients who have received neoadjuvant radiotherapy in combination with ELAPE.

A variety of alternatives to primary closure have been proposed in order to reconstruct the pelvic floor and to reduce the wound healing problems after APE. These procedures include omental pedicle flaps (omentoplasty), different local rotational musculocutaneous flaps, and biologic mesh interposition. Several reports using the rectus abduminus, gluteus maximus, or gracilis musculocutaneous flaps have been published.[38,39] In recent years, some experience with biologic mesh reconstruction of the pelvic floor has also been reported. This option seems feasible with a reasonable complication rate.[40] The published experience of different methods to reconstruct the pelvic floor, however, is still limited and based only on small cohort studies. A recent review of articles on the reconstruction of the perineum after ELAPE compared 255 patients undergoing flap repair with 85 patients undergoing biologic mesh repair and found no significant difference in the rates of perineal wound complications or perineal hernia formation.[41]

Currently, there is no standard solution for pelvic floor reconstruction after APE and the method must be tailored to patients and extent of excision. Thus, primary closure is almost always appropriate after an intersphincteric APE whereas some kind of mesh or flap reconstruction is often used after an ELAPE. After an ischioanal APE a flap reconstruction is almost always necessary, especially if the excision of skin has been extensive. It is recommended to assess each patient carefully before surgery to determine the suitable type of pelvic floor reconstruction and to establish collaboration with a plastic surgeon for reconstruction after the more wide excisions.

SUMMARY

Although treatment results in rectal cancer have improved significantly during the past two decades, local control and survival after APE have not improved to the same degree as seen after AR. The reason is an increased risk of inadvertent bowel perforations and tumor-involved margins after APE compared with AR. The conventional synchronous combined APE has not been a standardized procedure; hence, oncological outcomes have varied considerably between different institution and in different reports. With the new concept of APE, based on well-defined anatomic structures, the procedure can be categorized as intersphincteric APE, ELAPE, and ischioanal APE. Indications for each procedure should be based on a thorough preoperative tumor staging and clinical assessment of the patient. There are controversies related to the necessary extent of pelvic floor removal, to the positioning of the patient, and to the optimal method of reconstruction of the pelvic floor and perineum. The key objective must be, however, to remove an intact specimen without perforation and with resection margins free from tumor cells, which leads to improved local control and survival. With the recent focus on low rectal cancer, including staging, neoadjuvant treatments, and improved surgery, this goal can probably be achieved.

REFERENCES

1. Miles WE. A method of performing abdomino-perineal excision for carcinoma of the rectum and of the terminal portion of the pelvic colon. Lancet 1908;2:1812–3.
2. Collins DC. End-results of the Miles' combined abdominoperineal resection versus the segmental anterior resection. A 25-year postoperative follow-up in 301 patients. Am J Proctol 1963;14:258–61.
3. Fick TE, Baeten CG, von Meyenfeldt MF, et al. Recurrence and survival after abdominoperineal and low anterior resection for rectal cancer without adjunctive therapy. Eur J Surg Oncol 1990;16:105–8.
4. Groves RA, Harrison RC. Carcinoma of the rectum and lower sigmoid colon: abdominoperineal or anterior resection? Can J Surg 1962;5:393–403.
5. Slanetz CA, Herter FP, Grinnell RS. Anterior resection versus abdominoperineal resection for cancer of the rectum and rectosigmoid: an anlysis of 524 cases. Am J Surg 1972;123:110–7.
6. Vandertoll DJ, Beahrs OH. Carcinoma of the rectum and low sigmoid. Evaluation of anterior resection in 1766 favourable lesions. Arch Surg 1965;90:793–8.
7. Schmitz RL, Nelson EA, Martin GB, et al. Synchronous (two-team) abdominoperineal resection of the rectum. AMA Arch Surg 1958;77(4):492–7.
8. Påhlman L, Glimelius B. Local recurrences after surgical treatment for rectal carcinoma. Acta Chir Scand 1984;150:331–5.
9. Kapiteijn E, Marijnen CA, Nagtegaal ID, et al. Preoperative radiotherapy combined with total mesorectal excision for resectable rectal cancer. N Engl J Med 2001;345(9):638–46.
10. Swedish Rectal Cancer Trial, Improved survival with preoperative radiotherapy in resectable rectal cancer. N Engl J Med 1997;336:980–7.
11. Heald RJ, Husband EM, Ryall RD. The mesorectum in rectal cancer surgery–the clue to pelvic recurrence? Br J Surg 1982;69(10):613–6.
12. MacFarlane JK, Ryall RD, Heald RJ. Mesorectal excision for rectal cancer. Lancet 1993;341:457–60.

13. Wibe A, Moller B, Norstein J, et al. A national strategic change in treatment policy for rectal cancer–implementation of total mesorectal excision as routine treatment in Norway. A national audit. Dis Colon Rectum 2002;45(7):857–66.
14. Martling AL, Holm T, Rutqvist LE, et al. Effect of a surgical training programme on outcome of rectal cancer in the County of Stockholm. Stockholm Colorectal Cancer Study Group, Basingstoke Bowel Cancer Research Project. Lancet 2000; 356(9224):93–6.
15. Wibe A, Syse A, Andersen E, et al. Oncological outcomes after total mesorectal excision for cure for cancer of the lower rectum: anterior vs. abdominoperineal resection. Dis Colon Rectum 2004;47(1):48–58.
16. Marr R, Birbeck K, Garvican J, et al. The modern abdominoperineal excision: the next challenge after total mesorectal excision. Ann Surg 2005;242(1):74–82.
17. den Dulk M, Putter H, Collette L, et al. The abdominoperineal resection itself is associated with an adverse outcome: The European experience based on a pooled analysis of five European randomised clinical trials on rectal cancer. Eur J Cancer 2009;45(7):1175–83.
18. Nagtegaal ID, van de Velde CJH, Marijnen van Krieken JHJM, et al. Low rectal cancer: a call for a change of approach in abdominoperineal resection. J Clin Oncol 2005;23(36):9257–64.
19. Eriksen MT, Wibe A, Syse A, et al. Inadvertent perforation during rectal cancer resection in Norway. Br J Surg 2004;91(2):210–6.
20. den Dulk M, Marijnen CA, Putter H, et al. Risk factors for adverse outcome in patients with rectal cancer treated with an abdominoperineal resection in the total mesorectal excision trial. Ann Surg 2007;246(1):83–90.
21. Pollack J, Holm T, Cedermark B, et al. Long-term effect of preoperative radiation therapy on anorectal function. Dis Colon Rectum 2006;49(3):345–52.
22. Morris E, Quirke P, Thomas JD, et al. Unacceptable variation in abdominoperineal excision rates for rectal cancer: time to intervene? Gut 2008;57(12):1690–7.
23. Moore TJ, Moran BJ. Precision surgery, precision terminology: the origins and meaning of ELAPE. Colorectal Dis 2012;14(10):1173–4.
24. Birbeck KF, Macklin CP, Tiffin NJ, et al. Rates of circumferential resection margin involvement vary between surgeons and predict outcomes in rectal cancer surgery. Ann Surg 2002;235(4):449–57.
25. Radcliffe A. Can the results of anorectal (abdominoperineal) resection be improved: are circumferential resection margins too often positive? Colorectal Dis 2006;8(3):160–7.
26. Shihab OC, Heald RJ, Holm T, et al. A pictorial description of extralevator abdominoperineal excision for low rectal cancer. Colorectal Dis 2012;14(10):e655–60.
27. Stelzner S, Holm T, Moran BJ, et al. Deep pelvic anatomy revisited for a description of crucial steps in extralevator abdominoperineal excision for rectal cancer. Dis Colon Rectum 2011;54(8):947–57.
28. Shihab OC, Moran BJ, Heald RJ, et al. MRI staging of low rectal cancer. Eur Radiol 2009;19(3):643–50.
29. Holm T, Ljung A, Haggmark T, et al. Extended abdominoperineal resection with gluteus maximus flap reconstruction of the pelvic floor for rectal cancer. Br J Surg 2007;94(2):232–8.
30. West NP, Anderin C, Smith KJ, et al. Multicentre experience with extralevator abdominoperineal excision for low rectal cancer. Br J Surg 2010;97(4):588–99.
31. Stelzner S, Koehler C, Stelzer J, et al. Extended abdominoperineal excision vs. standard abdominoperineal excision in rectal cancer–a systematic overview. Int J Colorectal Dis 2011;26(10):1227–40.

32. Asplund D, Haglind E, Angenete E. Outcome of extralevator abdominoperineal excision compared with standard surgery: results from a single centre. Colorectal Dis 2012;14(10):1191–6.

33. Mathis KL, Larson DW, Dozois EJ, et al. Outcomes following surgery without radiotherapy for rectal cancer. Br J Surg 2012;99(1):137–43.

34. Krishna A, Rickard MJ, Keshava A, et al. A comparison of published rates of resection margin involvement and intra-operative perforation between standard and 'cylindrical' abdominoperineal excision for low rectal cancer. Colorectal Dis 2013;15(1):57–65.

35. de Campos-Lobato LF, Stocchi L, Dietz DW, et al. Prone or lithotomy positioning during an abdominoperineal resection for rectal cancer results in comparable oncologic outcomes. Dis Colon Rectum 2011;54(8):939–46.

36. Martijnse IS, Dudink RL, West NP, et al. Focus on extralevator perineal dissection in supine position for low rectal cancer has led to better quality of surgery and oncologic outcome. Ann Surg Oncol 2012;19(3):786–93.

37. Bullard KM, Trudel JL, Baxter NN, et al. Primary perineal wound closure after pre-operative radiotherapy and abdominoperineal resection has a high incidence of wound failure. Dis Colon Rectum 2005;48(3):438–43.

38. Khoo AK, Skibber JM, Nabawi AS, et al. Indications for immediate tissue transfer for soft tissue reconstruction in visceral pelvic surgery. Surgery 2001;130(3):463–9.

39. Nisar PJ, Scott HJ. Myocutaneous flap reconstruction of the pelvis after abdominoperineal excision. Colorectal Dis 2009;11(8):806–16.

40. Christensen HK, Nerstrøm P, Tei T, et al. Perineal repair after extralevator abdominoperineal excision for low rectal cancer. Dis Colon Rectum 2011;54(6):711–7.

41. Foster JD, Pathak S, Smart NJ, et al. Reconstruction of the perineum following extralevator abdominoperineal excision for carcinoma of the lower rectum: a systematic review. Colorectal Dis 2012;14(9):1052–9.

Management of Complete Response After Chemoradiation in Rectal Cancer

Martin R. Weiser, MD[a],*, Regina Beets-Tan, MD[b],
Gerard Beets, MD[c]

KEYWORDS

- Rectal cancer • Complete clinical response • Non-operative management
- Neoadjuvant therapy

KEY POINTS

- Among rectal cancer patients treated with neoadjuvant chemoradiation, 15% to 30% achieve a pathologic complete response (pCR).
- Smaller and less advanced tumors are more likely to have a pCR than larger and more advanced tumors.
- A complete clinical response is denoted by involution of the tumor to a flat and pale scar, and can take 10 to 12 weeks to be achieved.
- Studies to date indicate that local recurrence after nonoperative management occur within 12 to 18 months of treatment and can be salvaged with surgery.
- Studies need to be completed to determine ideal patient selection, treatment sequencing, optimal assessment of response, and long-term surveillance strategies.

INTRODUCTION

When a pathology report returns stating that there is "no residual tumor" in a patient treated with neoadjuvant therapy and rectal resection, a clinician is confronted with two conflicting emotions. The dominant feeling is one of delight, because a complete response to chemoradiation is associated with excellent clinical prognosis: a reported 5-year survival rate of 85% to 90%.[1] There is also a troubling sense of frustration, however, and even regret. Did the major resection add anything valuable other than providing histologic proof of a complete response? Was the risk of complication—including alterations in bowel function and detriment in quality of life associated

[a] Department of Surgery, Memorial Sloan–Kettering Cancer Center, 1275 York Avenue, New York, NY 10065, USA; [b] Department of Radiology, Maastricht University Medical Center, Minderbroedersberg 4, 6211 LK, Maastricht, The Netherlands; [c] Department of Surgery, Maastricht University Medical Center, Minderbroedersberg 4, 6211 LK, Maastricht, The Netherlands
* Corresponding author.
E-mail address: weiser1@MSKCC.ORG

Surg Oncol Clin N Am 23 (2014) 113–125
http://dx.doi.org/10.1016/j.soc.2013.09.012
1055-3207/14/$ – see front matter © 2014 Elsevier Inc. All rights reserved.
surgonc.theclinics.com

with surgery—justified? The question has largely been hypothetical, because it has been nearly impossible to detect a complete response by any means other than resection. There is growing evidence, however, that a more selective approach to surgery after chemoradiation may be rational. Although once limited to those patients too infirm to tolerate operation, several studies have now described organ-sparing treatment, or rectal preservation, in patients with significant tumor response to chemoradiation. These include reports of completely nonoperative approaches and minimal surgical approaches, such as local excision of the primary tumor site. This review investigates the concept of the nonoperative approach, also known as organ preservation, deferred surgery, or watch and wait, to rectal cancer patients treated for cure who have had a significant response to neoadjuvant therapy.

DEFINING COMPLETE RESPONSE

A pCR is defined as absence of viable tumor on histologic examination of a total mesorectal excision (TME) resection specimen, and is denoted as ypT0N0. A clinical complete response (cCR) is less clearly defined and usually describes absence of tumor, as based on a combination of digital rectal examination and endoscopy.[2] Thus, there is significant subjectivity and even potential bias in determining a cCR.

To further complicate matters, pCR is influenced by the interval between chemoradiation and surgery. If surgery is performed close to the time of radiation, tumor cells may be identified on histology but may not be viable. Furthermore, with current technology, it is impossible to histologically evaluate more than a small fraction of tissue after resection. Arguably, the best definition of a true complete response is retrospective: a sustained long-term absence of local tumor regrowth after nonoperative treatment.

INTERPRETING THE LITERATURE

In an attempt to understand the growing literature on organ-conserving treatment of rectal cancer, reports on patients treated with chemotherapy and radiation without surgery can be categorized into three clinical scenarios. Each category has limitations, but adds insight into the organ-preserving approach and is worth evaluating:

1. Patients who are unable or unwilling to have rectal resection. This group includes patients who are unfit for major operation, refuse surgery, or have disease such that they are treated in a palliative setting.
2. Patients with early rectal cancer who would likely be cured with radical TME surgery but elect chemoradiation in an attempt to avoid surgery. In these patients, cure with organ preservation is the aim of treatment.
3. Patients with locally advanced rectal cancer for whom neoadjuvant treatment and TME are the accepted standard. Although organ preservation is not the aim, it has been offered as an alternative treatment to those patients who obtain an excellent response.

Scenario 1: Patients Unfit for/Unwilling to Undergo Major Surgery

This group includes patients who decline surgery or are not candidates for operation. Most of these patients are not surgical candidates due to high operative risk related to frailty and excess comorbidity or advanced primary or metastatic disease, precluding curative resection. The primary aim in these cases is most often local control rather than long-term survival. The aim of treatment is palliation. To facilitate these goals, many centers prefer to give a higher radiotherapy dose than is delivered in the neoadjuvant setting. The assessment of response, usually by clinical examination and/ or CT imaging, is imprecise because it is of no therapeutic consequence. Thus, retrospective analysis of the rate of complete response is not highly accurate, and comparing these reports is unreliable.

The largest series in the literature is from the Princess Margaret Hospital in Toronto, reporting retrospectively on 271 patients, treated from 1978 to 1997 with external beam radiation therapy doses ranging from 40 to 60 Gy.[3] A complete clinical response, defined as no gross tumor on endoscopy or digital rectal examination, was obtained in 30% of patients after a median time of 4 months. The local relapse rate was 78% after a median time of 18 months. Washington University in St. Louis reported on 199 patients treated from 1981 to 1995 with endocavitary contact radiotherapy, with or without external beam radiation, as primary therapy. These were patients of advanced age, with excessive comorbidity, or who refused to proceed with any resection requiring colostomy.[4] The local control rate in this series was 71% after a median follow-up of 70 months. A series from Lyon, France, reports on 63 patients with intermediate-size tumors, treated with radiotherapy alone from 1986 to 1998.[5] A high localized dose of radiation was obtained using a combination of endoluminal contact therapy and external beam and interstitial brachytherapy. The cCR rate was an impressive 92% at 2 months after treatment, with a local control rate of 63% at 54 months. A Polish series, which used high doses (55–70 Gy) of conformal radiotherapy, with or without chemotherapy, in primary inoperable and recurrent rectal cancer, noted a cCR of 39%.[6] In addition to these series, there are several smaller reports that mostly include patients with large and inoperable tumors treated with standard external beam radiotherapy, with or without chemotherapy.[7–9] The rate of complete clinical response in these series varied from 10% to 50%, indicating a heterogeneous group of tumors.

Although it is not easy to draw conclusions from these series, some observations can be made. First, the definition and assessment of clinical response in these patient cohorts is highly variable. Second, maximal response to radiation, with or without chemotherapy, can take up to 4 to 6 months. Finally, these series confirm the basic rule of radiotherapy: that cCR and long-term local control are more likely in the setting of higher doses and smaller tumors.

Scenario 2: Patients with Early Rectal Cancer

This group includes patients with clinically small and superficial tumors who are attempting to avoid radical surgery. Common approaches include local excision and/or radiation. Failure rates after local excision, transanal excision, and transanal endoscopic microsurgery (TEM) without radiation range from 5% to 20%.[10,11] Undetected and untreated locoregional metastasis is hypothesized to result in a significant proportion of local recurrences.[12] Pelvic radiation (external beam and contact) is an alternative approach with a potential to treat the primary tumor and locoregional lymph nodes. Described by Papillon in France in the 1950s, endocavitary contact therapy delivers repetitive high doses to the luminal surface of a small distal rectal tumor. The result in early tumors is impressive, with a recent review reporting long-term local control rates of 85% to 90% in more than 1000 patients with clinical T1N0 tumors.[13] The success has led investigators to use this approach to avoid major surgery in more advanced rectal cancers. In a 2008 review, Borschitz and colleagues[14] reported a long-term local recurrence rate of 7% in 237 cT2/3 tumors treated with chemoradiation and local excision; 22% of patients had a pCR, and recurrence rates were directly associated with residual disease: 0% for ypT0, 2% for ypT1, 7% for ypT2, and 21% for ypT3 tumors. A report from the United Kingdom describes 220 patients with early rectal cancer receiving a combination of internal (contact) and external radiotherapy and local excision, with curative intent; 10% of patients showed poor response and underwent immediate rescue surgery. Of the remaining 90%, only 10% had late local recurrence, indicating that rectal preservation is possible in a significant subset of patients.[15]

The common theme of these studies is that smaller tumors sustain greater response to chemoradiation. When considering all patients, major surgery may be avoidable in up to 50%. The dilemma remains, however: Does the benefit to patients who respond to chemoradiation and avoid surgery outweigh the added toxicity and potential of overtreatment? This cohort of small and early rectal cancers would have excellent prognosis if treated with surgery alone. Maximizing response to increase the proportion of patients that achieves a cCR and avoids surgery would make chemoradiation more attractive.

Scenario 3: Patients with Locally Advanced Rectal Cancer Treated with Neoadjuvant Chemoradiation and Planned Surgery

The largest series of patients in this category is reported in several articles by Habr-Gama and colleagues,[16–21] and was summarized in a recent overview.[22] These studies involve generally fit patients with mid- to distal rectal cancers, for which the standard treatment is radiation with concurrent fluoropyrimidine, followed by total mesorectal excision. If patients had a cCR that was sustained for a year, they were entered into the study and managed nonoperatively. The proportion of sustained cCRs was reportedly approximately 30%, suggesting that a substantial number of less advanced tumors were included. The largest study from the Sao Paulo group was reported in 2006 and includes 361 patients treated in two hospitals.[20] Of 122 patients who had an initial cCR, 23 underwent rescue surgery within a year for early recurrence. Of the remaining 99 patients with sustained cCRs, 5 developed isolated local recurrence and 1 developed local and distant recurrence. With a mean follow-up of 60 months, 5-year overall survival was 93% and disease-free survival was 85%. The most recent update in 2011 reported on 173 patients treated at one of these two Sao Paulo centers, and confirms the excellent results: 96% overall survival and 75% disease-free survival at 5 years, with a mean follow-up of 65 months.[21] Of the 67 patients (39%) who achieved an initial cCR, 8 (11%) recurred locally; all recurrences were endoluminal and amenable to curative salvage surgery. Nine underwent diagnostic local excision.

Other, smaller studies have reported their experiences with observation after chemoradiation for rectal cancer. A retrospective series from Memorial Sloan–Kettering Cancer Center reported on 32 patients who achieved a cCR and were managed nonoperatively.[23] All patients were initially diagnosed with stage III disease or had a distal T2 tumor. Patients who declined surgery were older, had comorbidity, and/or had a strong desire to avoid the long-term morbidity associated with major surgery. After a median follow-up of 28 months, 6 patients suffered a local recurrence (5 endoluminal and 1 nodal), all within 14 months. The 3 patients with isolated local recurrence remain disease-free after salvage surgery. The overall survival rate was 96%, and similar to a comparison group of 57 patients with a pCR undergoing surgery.

A prospective series from Maastricht in the Netherlands described 21 patients with a cCR who were managed nonoperatively.[24] With a median follow-up of 25 months, there was only 1 patient with an isolated local recurrence (after 22 months), which was amenable to salvage surgery. This compared well with a group of patients who had pCR after major surgery. As expected, there were fewer stomas and better bowel function after organ-preserving treatment. In this series, modern MRI techniques played an important role in patient selection and follow-up.

Another retrospective study from India reported on 33 patients who achieved a cCR, of a cohort of 291 (11%) patients with locally advanced or very distal rectal cancer treated with neoadjuvant therapy.[25] Response was assessed by digital rectal examination and sigmoidoscopy at 4 to 6 weeks, and the definition of cCR allowed for minimal induration or mucosal irregularity; 23 of the 33 patients with cCR chose a watch-and-wait policy, the majority because of a wish to avoid a permanent stoma. Seven patients (30%) had local recurrence, 5 of these within the first year. A smaller series from the United Kingdom evaluated 49 patients with locally advanced rectal cancer treated with neoadjuvant therapy. Of the 6 patients with a cCR who opted to avoid surgery, none has recurred.[26]

In contrast to these studies reporting good outcomes, two older studies from another center in Sao Paulo noted high rates of local recurrence after nonoperative management in a small number of patients with cCR after chemoradiation (with and without brachytherapy) for locally advanced distal rectal cancer.[27,28] The reason for these divergent results is unknown, but may be a result of patient selection. Similar to other series, however, a majority of local recurrences were identified within the first year.

The use of transanal excision of the primary site after neoadjuvant therapy, in order to help identify cCR, was examined in a study of 174 patients from Israel.[29] All patients had locally advanced cancers of the mid- and lower rectum that responded well to neoadjuvant therapy. Digital examination, proctoscopy, and endorectal ultrasound identified 68 patients (39%) with possible cCR; 31 underwent local excision, yielding 23 with ypT0NX. All other patients underwent a major resection. With a long follow-up of 87 months, there were no local recurrences. Although this may constitute a compelling argument for using local excision to help identify cCR after chemoradiation, the approach is not without complications, including delayed healing and extended perioperative discomfort.[30]

Although the studies are heterogenous, with varying inclusion criteria, definitions of cCR, and modes of follow-up, some common themes exist. Recurrence after cCR most often presents within the first year. Salvage appears possible in the majority of cases. At this juncture, however, it must still be assumed that improvement in quality of life via nonoperative strategies is a trade-off, associated with some degree of increased oncologic risk. Many experts have recently written reviews and commentaries advising caution, noting that it is too early to propose nonoperative management as a standard treatment.[22,31–34]

ASSESSING RESPONSE TO CHEMORADIATION

Clearly, the Achilles' heel of any rectum-preserving approach is assessment of response. Only after improving the accuracy of response measurement can the benefit of a nonoperative approach be fully realized. Surgeons and radiotherapists who have been treating patients nonoperatively generally agree that there should be no stenosis, residual nodule, or even superficial ulceration on endoscopy or digital rectal examination.[2,23,24,35] A slight thickening of the bowel wall on palpation or some increased stiffness on endoscopy is compatible with fibrosis, and is not necessarily a sign of residual tumor. The best definition is provided in an article by Habr-Gama and colleagues,[2] which depicts the typical white scar with telangiectasis that often accompanies a complete response. Few studies have tried to establish the accuracy of these clinical findings. One study evaluated digital rectal examination immediately preceding a resection and found that only 21% of pCRs were detected, without any false-positive pCRs; the investigators attributed this underestimation of response to local inflammation and fibrosis interpreted as tumor remnant.[36] Although a positive biopsy is proof of residual tumor, a negative biopsy may be a false negative and cannot be relied on to exclude persistent disease.[37] Although local excision can accurately assess residual disease in the rectal wall, it is associated with significant morbidity after chemoradiation.[30] Furthermore, this approach does not include assessment of locoregional lymph nodes, which can harbor disease in 5% to 10% of patients with no residual rectal wall malignancy (ypT0N1).[38]

Given the subjective nature of digital examination and endoscopy, other modalities are needed to assess residual disease after neoadjuvant therapy for rectal cancer. Modern imaging techniques are able to measure rectal wall lesions and lymph nodes, but restaging after chemoradiation remains challenging.

Restaging with endorectal ultrasound yields variable and generally disappointing rates of accuracy in assessing T stage, ranging from 40% to 75%.[39–43] The largest study, by Pastor and colleagues,[43] reported a predictive value of only 47% in assessment of complete response. Endorectal ultrasound was especially limited in detecting small tumor remnants within fibrotic tissue. At the same time, 76% of ypT0 tumors were overstaged because of difficulties in interpreting fibrosis. This same study showed an accuracy of 75% for nodal restaging, similar to that shown in smaller, earlier studies.[43] The low sensitivity (39%) and high specificity (91%) in the study group led to a negative predictive value of 72%, implying that, in an organ-preserving approach, endorectal ultrasound cannot detect lymph nodes containing minimal residual disease.

CT–positron emission tomography (PET) accurately measures tumor response after neoadjuvant therapy in many malignancies; however, it has been less useful in the evaluation of rectal cancer and does not seem accurate enough to guide treatment. Most studies have compared the standardized uptake value (SUV) before with the SUV at variable intervals after completion of chemoradiotherapy, correlating this with a histologic measure of response. A meta-analysis published in 2012, including 28 studies with 1204 patients, reported 78% sensitivity and 62% specificity for prediction of response with PET after chemoradiation, and a sensitivity of 86% and specificity of 80% with PET during chemoradiation.[44] Since publication of this meta-analysis, at least 15 additional reports have generally confirmed that change in PET SUV correlates well with response. The problem is that the histologic measure of response is not uniform, and, in most studies, complete responses are grouped together with near-complete responses, rendering the results less applicable to the prediction and assessment of a complete response. This is well illustrated by a recent large study reported by Guillem and colleagues[45] that specifically focused on assessment of complete response, demonstrating a disappointingly low area under the curve in the receiver operating characteristic curve of 0.64, and a sensitivity of 54%, with a specificity of 66%. On its own, this level of accuracy is considered insufficient, and the added value of CT-PET to endoscopy and axial imaging in the management of clinical complete responders is limited using current technology.

Most recently, attention has been directed to MRI and functional MRI. A pooled analysis of 33 studies reported on restaging with MRI in 1556 patients.[46] For ypT stage, the overall mean sensitivity was 50%, with a specificity of 91%. Subgroup analyses showed only 19% sensitivity, with 94% specificity, for the assessment of ypT0. This poor performance was again mainly due to difficulties in interpretation due to fibrosis. Conventional MRI cannot differentiate between fibrosis with and without tumor remnants, and tends to overestimate residual tumor. When volumetric changes are combined with morphologic features, however, the accuracy of MRI assessment of ypT0 and ypT0-2 tumors increases from 50% to 80% to 90%.[47–49] The additional use of functional MRI, such as diffusion-weighted imaging and dynamic contrast-enhanced MRI, appears to further improve identification of a complete response by raising the sensitivity to 84% while keeping specificity at 85%.[46] Primary nodal staging is only moderately accurate, with sensitivities and specificities of 55% to 75%, because of limitations in detecting small metastatic foci. Examples are shown in **Figs. 1** and **2**. There is some evidence, however, that with new MRI techniques this could improve to 70% to 85%.[50–52] With respect to nodal restaging, a recent meta-analysis shows a sensitivity of 77% and a specificity of 60%.[46] With a low prevalence of involved nodes after chemoradiation, this results in a negative predictive value of 80% to 90%. It is the authors' experience that MRI nodal restaging is more accurate than primary staging, because change in node size after treatment is informative.[53,54]

A confounding factor in these studies is the lack of standardization in the timing of examination after neoadjuvant therapy. Response continues over time, and the number of patients with a pCR increases with a longer interval after chemoradiation.[55,56] Thus, the Sao Paulo group routinely assesses patients after an interval of at least 8 weeks. More recent studies indicate that it may be safe to continue observation for up to 12 weeks.[57]

FUTURE STUDIES

A prospective randomized trial comparing nonoperative management to standard therapy, including surgery, would be optimal in assessing the efficacy and safety of

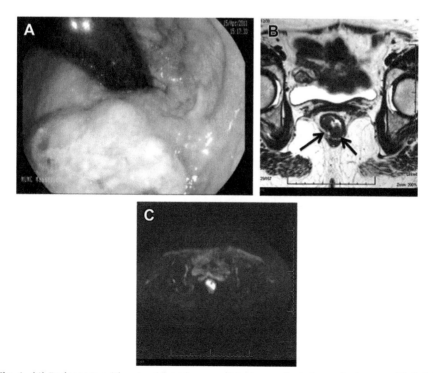

Fig. 1. (*A*) Endoscopy with retrovision shows a distal tumor, just above the levator. (*B*) Axial MRI of the posteriorly located rectal cancer (*arrows*). (*C*) Corresponding diffusion-weighted imaging showing a high tumor signal.

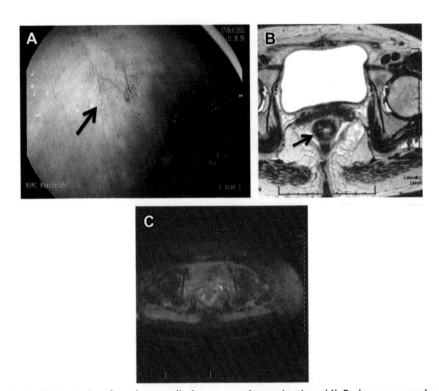

Fig. 2. Eight weeks after chemoradiation, a rectal examination. (*A*) Endoscopy reveals a normal rectal wall with at endoscopy a flat whitish scar with some teleangiectasis (*arrow*), typical for a complete response. (*B*) On MRI, the tumor has disappeared and is replaced by some fibrotic changes in the bowel wall (*arrow*). (*C*) Corresponding diffusion-weighted imaging shows a complete disappearance of tumor signal. There are no suspicious nodes in the mesorectum (images not shown). The patient opted for a nonoperative management and remains free of disease 3 years later.

nonoperative management. Accrual might be challenging, because many patients might resist random assignment to radical surgery when presented with the alternative option of rectal preservation. High-quality phase II trials are more likely to be acceptable to patients, given the interest many express in organ-preserving therapy. The observations of Smith and colleagues[23] are especially useful when considering such a trial. Highly stringent criteria to assess cCR must be developed based on digital examination and endoscopy. Dynamic MRI holds promise for assisting in assessment of response and should be studied further. Patients should be assessed 6 to 8 weeks after treatment, to identify those who have had a suboptimal response so that they may proceed with surgery. Those patients who are responding well but still demonstrate small areas of induration, nodularity, or ulceration should be reassessed at 10 to 12 weeks after chemoradiation, to allow for continued tumor regression to a bland, flat scar. Patients who have achieved a convincing cCR (ie, an endoscopic pale, flat scar [with or without telangiectasias]), may begin post-treatment monitoring or proceed with adjuvant chemotherapy. The role of biopsy is not clear. Surface biopsies are rarely helpful and often misleading, and transanal excision is associated with significant morbidity.

Once patients are designated as having a cCR, the next critical aspect of nonoperative management is close monitoring for local tumor recurrence. The data demonstrate that a majority of local relapses occur within 12 to 18 months. Patients should be clinically and endoscopically examined at regular intervals. It seems reasonable to examine patients every 3 to 4 months for the first 12 to 18 months, and then every 6 to 8 months thereafter. Again, the role of dynamic MRI must be defined, but it has the potential to aid in surveillance.

As trials are designed, pretreatment biopsies must be included for molecular correlate studies. A molecular signature associated with complete response (or nonresponse) would enrich study cohorts suitable for nonoperative management.

SUMMARY

One of the emerging themes in modern rectal cancer treatment is improving quality of life by avoiding overtreatment. Traditionally, therapy for locally advanced rectal cancer has been trimodal: chemotherapy, radiation, and surgery. The oncologic outcome is generally good, with low rates of local recurrence; however, there is a tradeoff with regard to morbidity, including bowel, urinary, and sexual dysfunction.[58] Is such intensive therapy needed for all stage II and III rectal cancer patients? Can some of the treatment be eliminated? The Preoperative Radiation or Selective Preoperative Radiation and Evaluation before Chemotherapy and Total Mesorectal Excision (PROSPECT) (N1048) trial asks whether pelvic radiotherapy can be used selectively rather than uniformly. Another approach is to eliminate surgery for those patients who respond well to neoadjuvant chemoradiation. The current studies indicate that 15% to 30% of patients have a pCR, and may be candidates for nonoperative management. Local recurrences in those who have deferred surgery generally occur within 12 to 18 months of completing therapy, and most appear to be salvageable. It must be remembered, however, that until the long-term durability of the nonoperative approach can be proven, surgery remains the standard of care. Well-designed prospective studies are necessary to answer the many remaining questions, including patient selection, sequencing of treatment, optimal assessment of response, and long-term surveillance.

REFERENCES

1. Quah HM, Chou JF, Gonen M, et al. Pathologic stage is most prognostic of disease-free survival in locally advanced rectal cancer patients after preoperative chemoradiation. Cancer 2008;113(1):57–64.
2. Habr-Gama A, Perez O, Wynn G, et al. Complete clinical response after neoadjuvant chemoradiation therapy for distal rectal cancer: characterization of clinical and endoscopic findings for standardization. Dis Colon Rectum 2010; 53(12):1692–8.
3. Wang Y, Cummings B, Catton P, et al. Primary radical external beam radiotherapy of rectal adenocarcinoma: long term outcome of 271 patients. Radiother Oncol 2005;77(2):126–32.
4. Aumock A, Birnbaum EH, Fleshman JW, et al. Treatment of rectal adenocarcinoma with endocavitary and external beam radiotherapy: results for 199 patients with localized tumors. Int J Radiat Oncol Biol Phys 2001;51(2):363–70.
5. Gerard JP, Chapet O, Ramaioli A, et al. Long-term control of T2-T3 rectal adenocarcinoma with radiotherapy alone. Int J Radiat Oncol Biol Phys 2002;54(1): 142–9.

6. Sprawka A, Pietrzak L, Garmol D, et al. Definitive radical external beam radiotherapy for rectal cancer: evaluation of local effectiveness and risk of late small bowel damage. Acta Oncol 2013;52(4):816–23.

7. Hughes R, Harrison M, Glynne-Jones R. Could a wait and see policy be justified in T3/4 rectal cancers after chemo-radiotherapy? Acta Oncol 2010;49(3):378–81.

8. Lim L, Chao M, Shapiro J, et al. Long-term outcomes of patients with localized rectal cancer treated with chemoradiation or radiotherapy alone because of medical inoperability or patient refusal. Dis Colon Rectum 2007;50(12): 2032–9.

9. Overgaard M, Bertelsen K, Dalmark M, et al. A randomized feasibility study evaluating the effect of radiotherapy alone or combined with 5-fluorouracil in the treatment of locally recurrent or inoperable colorectal carcinoma. Acta Oncol 1993;32(5):547–53.

10. You YN. Local excision: is it an adequate substitute for radical resection in t1/t2 patients? Semin Radiat Oncol 2011;21(3):178–84.

11. Bach SP, Hill J, Monson JR, et al. A predictive model for local recurrence after transanal endoscopic microsurgery for rectal cancer. Br J Surg 2009;96(3): 280–90.

12. Landmann RG, Wong WD, Hoepfl J, et al. Limitations of early rectal cancer nodal staging may explain failure after local excision. Dis Colon Rectum 2007; 50(10):1520–5.

13. Gerard JP, Romestaing P, Chapet O. Radiotherapy alone in the curative treatment of rectal carcinoma. Lancet Oncol 2003;4(3):158–66.

14. Borschitz T, Wachtlin D, Mohler M, et al. Neoadjuvant chemoradiation and local excision for T2-3 rectal cancer. Ann Surg Oncol 2008;15(3):712–20.

15. Sun Myint A, Grieve RJ, McDonald AC, et al. Combined modality treatment of early rectal cancer: the UK experience. Clin Oncol (R Coll Radiol) 2007;19(9): 674–81.

16. Habr-Gama A. Assessment and management of the complete clinical response of rectal cancer to chemoradiotherapy. Colorectal Dis 2006;8(Suppl 3):21–4.

17. Habr-Gama A, de Souza PM, Ribeiro U Jr, et al. Low rectal cancer: impact of radiation and chemotherapy on surgical treatment. Dis Colon Rectum 1998; 41(9):1087–96.

18. Habr-Gama A, Perez RO, Nadalin W, et al. Long-term results of preoperative chemoradiation for distal rectal cancer correlation between final stage and survival. J Gastrointest Surg 2005;9(1):90–9 [discussion: 99–101].

19. Habr-Gama A, Perez RO, Nadalin W, et al. Operative versus nonoperative treatment for stage 0 distal rectal cancer following chemoradiation therapy: long-term results. Ann Surg 2004;240(4):711–7 [discussion: 717–8].

20. Habr-Gama A, Perez RO, Proscurshim I, et al. Patterns of failure and survival for nonoperative treatment of stage c0 distal rectal cancer following neoadjuvant chemoradiation therapy. J Gastrointest Surg 2006;10(10):1319–28 [discussion: 1328–9].

21. Habr-Gama A, Perez RO, Sao Juliao GP, et al. Nonoperative approaches to rectal cancer: a critical evaluation. Semin Radiat Oncol 2011;21(3):234–9.

22. Glynne-Jones R, Hughes R. Critical appraisal of the 'wait and see' approach in rectal cancer for clinical complete responders after chemoradiation. Br J Surg 2012;99(7):897–909.

23. Smith JD, Ruby JA, Goodman KA, et al. Nonoperative management of rectal cancer with complete clinical response after neoadjuvant therapy. Ann Surg 2012;256(6):965–72.

24. Maas M, Beets-Tan RG, Lambregts DM, et al. Wait-and-see policy for clinical complete responders after chemoradiation for rectal cancer. J Clin Oncol 2011;29(35):4633–40.
25. Seshadri RA, Kondaveeti SS, Jayanand SB, et al. Complete clinical response to neoadjuvant chemoradiation in rectal cancers: can surgery be avoided? Hepatogastroenterology 2013;60(123):410–4.
26. Dalton RS, Velineni R, Osborne ME, et al. A single-centre experience of chemoradiotherapy for rectal cancer: is there potential for nonoperative management? Colorectal Dis 2012;14(5):567–71.
27. Nakagawa WT, Rossi BM, de O Ferreira F, et al. Chemoradiation instead of surgery to treat mid and low rectal tumors: is it safe? Ann Surg Oncol 2002;9(6):568–73.
28. Rossi BM, Nakagawa WT, Novaes PE, et al. Radiation and chemotherapy instead of surgery for low infiltrative rectal adenocarcinoma: a prospective trial. Ann Surg Oncol 1998;5(2):113–8.
29. Issa N, Murninkas A, Powsner E, et al. Long-term outcome of local excision after complete pathological response to neoadjuvant chemoradiation therapy for rectal cancer. World J Surg 2012;36(10):2481–7.
30. Garcia-Aguilar J, Shi Q, Thomas CR Jr, et al. A phase II trial of neoadjuvant chemoradiation and local excision for T2N0 rectal cancer: preliminary results of the ACOSOG Z6041 trial. Ann Surg Oncol 2012;19(2):384–91.
31. Smith FM, Waldron D, Winter DC. Rectum-conserving surgery in the era of chemoradiotherapy. Br J Surg 2010;97(12):1752–64.
32. Hingorani M, Hartley JE, Greenman J, et al. Avoiding radical surgery after preoperative chemoradiotherapy: a possible therapeutic option in rectal cancer? Acta Oncol 2012;51(3):275–84.
33. Singh-Ranger G, Kumar D. Current concepts in the non-operative management of rectal cancer after neoadjuvant chemoradiation. Anticancer Res 2011;31(5):1795–800.
34. O'Neill BD, Brown G, Heald RJ, et al. Non-operative treatment after neoadjuvant chemoradiotherapy for rectal cancer. Lancet Oncol 2007;8(7):625–33.
35. Ortholan C, Romestaing P, Chapet O, et al. Correlation in rectal cancer between clinical tumor response after neoadjuvant radiotherapy and sphincter or organ preservation: 10-year results of the Lyon R 96-02 randomized trial. Int J Radiat Oncol Biol Phys 2012;83(2):e165–71.
36. Guillem JG, Chessin DB, Shia J, et al. Clinical examination following preoperative chemoradiation for rectal cancer is not a reliable surrogate end point. J Clin Oncol 2005;23(15):3475–9.
37. Maretto I, Pomerri F, Pucciarelli S, et al. The potential of restaging in the prediction of pathologic response after preoperative chemoradiotherapy for rectal cancer. Ann Surg Oncol 2007;14(2):455–61.
38. Maas M, Nelemans PJ, Valentini V, et al. Long-term outcome in patients with a pathological complete response after chemoradiation for rectal cancer: a pooled analysis of individual patient data. Lancet Oncol 2010;11(9):835–44.
39. Vanagunas A, Lin DE, Stryker SJ. Accuracy of endoscopic ultrasound for restaging rectal cancer following neoadjuvant chemoradiation therapy. Am J Gastroenterol 2004;99(1):109–12.
40. Napoleon B, Pujol B, Berger F, et al. Accuracy of endosonography in the staging of rectal cancer treated by radiotherapy. Br J Surg 1991;78(7):785–8.
41. Radovanovic Z, Breberina M, Petrovic T, et al. Accuracy of endorectal ultrasonography in staging locally advanced rectal cancer after preoperative chemoradiation. Surg Endosc 2008;22(11):2412–5.

42. Huh JW, Park YA, Jung EJ, et al. Accuracy of endorectal ultrasonography and computed tomography for restaging rectal cancer after preoperative chemoradiation. J Am Coll Surg 2008;207(1):7–12.

43. Pastor C, Subtil JC, Sola J, et al. Accuracy of endoscopic ultrasound to assess tumor response after neoadjuvant treatment in rectal cancer: can we trust the findings? Dis Colon Rectum 2011;54(9):1141–6.

44. Zhang C, Tong J, Sun X, et al. 18F-FDG-PET evaluation of treatment response to neo-adjuvant therapy in patients with locally advanced rectal cancer: a meta-analysis. Int J Cancer 2012;131(11):2604–11.

45. Guillem JG, Ruby JA, Leibold T, et al. Neither FDG-PET nor CT can distinguish between a pathological complete response and an incomplete response after neoadjuvant chemoradiation in locally advanced rectal cancer: a prospective study. Ann Surg 2013;258(2):289–95.

46. van der Paardt MP, Zagers MB, Beets-Tan RG, et al. Patients who undergo preoperative chemoradiotherapy for locally advanced rectal cancer restaged by using diagnostic MR imaging: a systematic review and meta-analysis. Radiology 2013;269(1):101–12.

47. Barbaro B, Fiorucci C, Tebala C, et al. Locally advanced rectal cancer: MR imaging in prediction of response after preoperative chemotherapy and radiation therapy. Radiology 2009;250(3):730–9.

48. Dresen RC, Beets GL, Rutten HJ, et al. Locally advanced rectal cancer: MR imaging for restaging after neoadjuvant radiation therapy with concomitant chemotherapy. Part I. Are we able to predict tumor confined to the rectal wall? Radiology 2009;252(1):71–80.

49. Curvo-Semedo L, Lambregts DM, Maas M, et al. Rectal cancer: assessment of complete response to preoperative combined radiation therapy with chemotherapy–conventional MR volumetry versus diffusion-weighted MR imaging. Radiology 2011;260(3):734–43.

50. Lahaye MJ, Engelen SM, Nelemans PJ, et al. Imaging for predicting the risk factors–the circumferential resection margin and nodal disease–of local recurrence in rectal cancer: a meta-analysis. Semin Ultrasound CT MR 2005;26(4):259–68.

51. Bipat S, Glas AS, Slors FJ, et al. Rectal cancer: local staging and assessment of lymph node involvement with endoluminal US, CT, and MR imaging–a meta-analysis. Radiology 2004;232(3):773–83.

52. Beets-Tan RG. Pretreatment MRI of lymph nodes in rectal cancer: an opinion-based review. Colorectal Dis 2013;15(7):781–4.

53. Lambregts DM, Beets GL, Maas M, et al. Accuracy of gadofosveset-enhanced MRI for nodal staging and restaging in rectal cancer. Ann Surg 2011;253(3):539–45.

54. Lambregts DM, Maas M, Riedl RG, et al. Value of ADC measurements for nodal staging after chemoradiation in locally advanced rectal cancer-a per lesion validation study. Eur Radiol 2011;21(2):265–73.

55. Moore HG, Gittleman AE, Minsky BD, et al. Rate of pathologic complete response with increased interval between preoperative combined modality therapy and rectal cancer resection. Dis Colon Rectum 2004;47(3):279–86.

56. Kalady MF, de Campos-Lobato LF, Stocchi L, et al. Predictive factors of pathologic complete response after neoadjuvant chemoradiation for rectal cancer. Ann Surg 2009;250(4):582–9.

57. Garcia-Aguilar J, Smith DD, Avila K, et al, Timing of Rectal Cancer Response to Chemoradiation Consortium. Optimal timing of surgery after chemoradiation for

advanced rectal cancer: preliminary results of a multicenter, nonrandomized phase II prospective trial. Ann Surg 2011;254(1):97–102.

58. Loos M, Quentmeier P, Schuster T, et al. Effect of preoperative radio(chemo) therapy on long-term functional outcome in rectal cancer patients: a systematic review and meta-analysis. Ann Surg Oncol 2013;20(6):1816–28.

Functional Consequences of Colorectal Cancer Management

Daniel Fish, MD, Larissa K. Temple, MD, FASC, FRCS(C)*

KEYWORDS

- Colorectal cancer • Bowel dysfunction • Urinary dysfunction • Sexual dysfunction
- Impotence • Incontinence • Urgency • Pouch

KEY POINTS

- Post-treatment dysfunction is prevalent and often severe in rectal cancer patients. Colon cancer patients are comparatively spared. The literature is difficult to assimilate, and, in general, data regarding many factors potentially affecting function are scarce.
- Bowel dysfunction after rectal cancer treatment is closely related to tumor height, which determines preservation of the anal sphincters and rectal capacity. It is also affected by pouch reconstruction and radiotherapy.
- Sexual dysfunction after rectal cancer treatment remains poorly understood, due in part to insufficient measurement of preoperative function and psychosocial confounders. It is worse with increasing age and low-lying tumors and after abdominoperineal resection (APR), ostomy, nerve injury, or radiotherapy.
- Urinary dysfunction after rectal cancer treatment remains poorly understood. There are multiple types of urinary dysfunction. It is worse with increasing age, female gender, advanced stage tumors, nerve injury, and APR.
- Standardization of measurement using validated instruments is needed to improve understanding of dysfunction. Reduction of toxicity in the treatment paradigm and interventions, such as physical therapy, pharmacologic therapy, and sacral neuromodulation, may help reduce the prevalence and severity of post-treatment dysfunction.

INTRODUCTION

Oncologic outcomes in patients with colorectal cancer have improved significantly within the past decade. Although effective, the treatment of colorectal cancer has a long-term impact on patients' bowel, bladder, and sexual functions. Post-treatment dysfunction affects patients socially and psychologically. The functional consequences of colorectal cancer treatment and post-treatment quality of life (QOL) have become increasingly important in clinical practice and research. Understanding the scope,

The authors have nothing to disclose.
Section of Colorectal Service, Department of Surgery, Memorial Sloan-Kettering Cancer Center, 1275 York Avenue, New York, NY 10065, USA
* Corresponding author.
E-mail address: templel@mskcc.org

severity, and prevalence of the functional consequences of therapy is integral to setting appropriate patient expectations, evaluating new therapies, and developing novel methods of function preservation and restoration. This article discusses bowel, sexual, and bladder functions in patients undergoing treatment of colon and rectal cancer.

BOWEL FUNCTION

Bowel dysfunction is a common side effect of treatment of colorectal cancer. Although the chemotherapeutic agents commonly used have minimal gastrointestinal toxicity, most patients report experiencing some changes to bowel function after treatment.[1] The extent of recovery after therapy largely depends on the location of the tumor and the type of resection.

Colon Cancer

After treatment of colon cancer, patients may experience mild bowel dysfunction, varying in intensity and manifestation depending on the colonic segment that was resected. In a comparison survey of a retrospective population, right hemicolectomy resulted in higher frequency, whereas left hemicolectomy resulted in greater difficulty emptying.[2] After sigmoid colectomy, some patients experience increased frequency, incomplete emptying, and difficulty evacuating, at rates of 5%, 32%, and 32%, respectively.[3] Although some dysfunction exists after surgery for colon cancer, proctectomy results in significantly more functional defects.[2] Regardless, it is important to discuss potential alterations in bowel function in patients being treated for colon cancer, especially those with sigmoid tumors.

Rectal Cancer

Most patients with rectal cancer seek a sphincter-preserving option and are reluctant to accept a permanent stoma. With improved surgical techniques, neoadjuvant therapy, and more limited distal surgical margins, sphincter-preserving surgery is more commonly offered. Nationally, sphincter preservation rates have increased.[4] At specialty centers, sphincter preservation is common even for tumors located less than 4 cm from the anal verge.[5] Many single-center studies report that intersphincteric resections (ISRs) with hand-sewn anastomoses for very low tumors result in equivalent oncologic outcomes.[6] These developments heighten the importance of understanding the impact of therapy on bowel function.

With sphincter preservation increasing, surgeons are investing significant clinical and research energy on the management of post-treatment bowel function. In a recent report, 56% of patients undergoing total mesorectal excision (TME) low anterior resection (LAR) met the criteria for LAR syndrome, significant incontinence, or increased frequency, but these figures improved to 28% by 1 year postoperation.[7] Years after sphincter-preserving LAR, however, 37% of patients report disappointment with their bowel function and 27% report their symptoms as severe, the most common symptoms being incomplete evacuation, clustering, food affecting frequency, unformed stool, and gas incontinence.[8] Many patient factors, tumor factors, and treatment factors affect function, and these are discussed.

Patient Factors

Age

Although bowel dysfunction is more prevalent in the general elderly population, age does not significantly affect the incidence of post-treatment bowel dysfunction.[7,9–11] Some research has found that younger patients report worse function,[12] possibly because it affects their QOL more profoundly. Although elderly patients score slightly worse on functional and role domains of QOL metrics, worsened functional outcomes have not been documented in older patients. Further systematic study is needed.

Gender

Whether there is a gender difference in bowel dysfunction after therapy remains unclear. Data comparing bowel function after rectal cancer therapy by gender are mixed, with some studies reporting greater dysfunction in women,[12] some reporting greater dysfunction in men,[13] and some reporting no difference.[14] It is possible that preexisting subclinical sphincter injuries exist more commonly in women due to childbirth, predisposing women to worse postoperative bowel function. To date, however, there have been mixed data supporting or refuting differences in function based on gender.

Preoperative function

Preoperative bowel function should intuitively play a role in post-treatment bowel function. In assessment for sphincter-preservation, an understanding of each patient's current function is crucial to making appropriate recommendations. Pretreatment function has not been well measured, however, and further research is necessary to determine the magnitude of this relationship.

Tumor Factors

Tumor level

The level of tumor and its unique effect on function is under-reported. Using the level of the anastomosis as a surrogate for tumor height, tumor level appears to be one of the most important factors affecting post-treatment bowel function. Lower tumors require more extensive and challenging dissection, which incurs an elevated risk of injury to the autonomic nerves, pelvic floor, and anal sphincter. Many studies have confirmed the relevance of anastomotic height to subsequent function, and some have found the effect so strong as to be the only predictor of dysfunction[15,16] or the best predictor of postoperative improvement.[7] Frequency, incontinence, emptying problems, and difficulty discriminating stool from gas increase significantly if the anastomosis is located 3 to 7 cm from the anal verge.[17,18] ISRs required for low tumors may pose a particularly high risk of incontinence, embarrassment, and reliance on medication[19]; meta-analysis demonstrates significant rates of incontinence (49%), soiling (29%), urgency (18%), and medication reliance (18%) after ISR.[20] Tumor proximity to the anal verge and subsequent anastomotic height are key determinants of postoperative bowel function and must be considered in patient counseling and treatment planning.

Tumor stage

The effect of stage on bowel function is difficult to separate from the effects of stage-specific treatments. As tumors become bulkier (ie, T4 lesions), the need to resect additional anatomic structures may have a further impact on functional outcomes. In patients with stage II or III tumors, however, it is difficult to isolate the impact of stage from other factors, such as radiation, and the unique affect of tumor stage on bowel function remains difficult to describe.

Treatment Factors

Open versus minimally invasive technique

Whether differences in visualization, tactile sensation, retraction, or maneuverability in open, laparoscopic, or robotic surgical approaches translate to differences in postoperative bowel function remains poorly understood. Several randomized studies have evaluated inpatient milestones, perioperative and longer-term oncologic outcomes associated with open versus laparoscopic rectal surgery, but no study has rigorously evaluated functional outcomes. Early data from the COLOR II trial suggest that no difference has been seen in functional outcomes at 12 months postoperatively,[21] but further research is needed. Data from the multicenter randomized ACOSOG Z6051 trial are awaited and may provide additional insight.

TME and non-TME approaches

TME is considered the gold standard for the surgical treatment of most rectal cancers, and modern functional outcomes are generally reported in patients who have undergone TME. In two instances, functional outcomes have been reported for nontraditional TME surgical procedures for rectal cancer.

Extended lateral pelvic lymph node dissection (ELND) in locally advanced cancer is not practiced routinely in North America but has been used more extensively in Asia. The literature on subsequent bowel function is limited but suggests that physiologic parameters of evacuation are not negatively affected.[22] This work is significantly confounded, however, by increased use of radiation, J pouch, and autonomic nerve dissection in patients requiring lymph node dissection.

Transanal endoscopic microsurgery (TEM) may be a viable excisional approach in select cases of rectal cancer. Although the data on functional outcomes are limited, and no direct comparison with proctectomy exists, TEM seems to produce good functional results, resulting in mild bowel dysfunction[23] that improves after 3 to 12 months and returns to baseline,[24] with maintenance of high QOL.[23,24] Given its favorable functional profile, transanal excision should be considered an option in oncologically appropriate cases, although further research is necessary.

Reconstructive techniques

Decisions regarding the method of restoring bowel continuity after proctectomy can significantly affect subsequent bowel function. Restorative methods are of particular importance to surgeons because of their discretionary nature and afford an opportunity to positively influence subsequent function. For this reason, many high-quality studies have been performed examining function after specific reconstructive techniques.

Hand-sewn versus stapled anastomosis

Restorative bowel anastomoses were traditionally performed using suture, but the development of complex bowel staplers have made stapled anastomoses increasingly popular, and their adoption has been facilitated by studies reporting similar function between hand-sewn and stapled anastomosis.[25] A recent randomized trial also found no difference in function.[26] In modern series, patients with hand-sewn anastomosis typically have worse function, but this is most likely due to the use of suture as a proxy for a very low anastomosis. Therefore, ease of anastomosis with suture or stapler is likely the best determinant of method.

Restorative pouches

The straight end-to-end anastomosis has been noted to result in significant frequency, urgency, and clustering, likely due to smaller capacity, distensibility, and increased peristaltic motility compared with native rectum.[27] Therefore, neorectal reconstructions, such as the side-to-end anastomosis, J pouch, and coloplasty pouches, have been devised in an attempt to better restore function, and several studies have evaluated their relative merits.

Many trials have found the J pouch functionally superior to the straight anastomosis. J pouch is associated with 50% fewer bowel movements[28–30] and less nocturnal frequency,[28] urgency,[29,31] incontinence,[29,32] clustering,[30] retention,[29] medication reliance,[29,30] need for dietary restriction,[30] difficulty with discrimination,[29] capacity, and compliance.[31] The superiority of the J pouch may increase with proximity to the anal verge[27,33]; thus, patients with anastomoses less than 4 cm from the anus may benefit most. These advantages last at least 18 months after surgery.[34] Data on longer-term outcomes are mixed. Some studies report equalization over time,[29] whereas others report continued superiority at 5 years. The J pouch balances storage and expulsion best when 5 to 6 cm in length,[35] and sigmoid and descending colon J pouches function equally well.[36] There are some reports of increased need for enemas with a pouch, especially pouches longer than 5 cm.[16,35] Overall, the J pouch seems to provide better function than straight anastomosis; however, construction of a J pouch is not always technically feasible.

Other pouch options exist. The transverse coloplasty pouch has shown functional equivalence to the J pouch in some randomized studies.[37–39] In a large, well-controlled randomized study, however, Fazio and colleagues[40] found it to have inferior functional results compared with the J pouch. Ho and colleagues[37] reported a high leak rate (16%) occurring at the antimesenteric side of the end-to-end anastomosis. Another option, the side-to-end anastomosis, requires less physical space and is easier to construct than the J pouch, with fewer staple lines. Side-to-end anastomosis has been shown to produce better functional outcomes than the straight end-to-end anastomosis[41] and similar results to the J pouch, although the J pouch demonstrated mildly better recovery of capacity[42] and better evacuation at 6 months.[43] Despite these data, the transverse coloplasty pouch and side-to-end anastomosis have not been as widely adopted as the J pouch.

In summary, all neorectal constructions seem to provide better function than the straight end-to-end anastomosis for at least the first 12 to 24 months postoperatively. The J pouch reconstruction seems associated with slightly better recovery than the side-to-end anastomosis but is more bulky. The J pouch produces fewer leaks, and likely better function, than the coloplasty pouch. Additional long-term outcome data are required in order for us to better understand the durability and function of various pouch reconstructions.

Diverting ileostomy

Although diverting ileostomy has been shown to decrease postoperative ileus,[44] reoperation,[45] anastomotic leak, and pelvic sepsis,[45–48] diversion has unclear effects on long-term function. Diversion has the potential to cause atrophy, stricture, or disuse colitis, which could affect longer-term postoperative bowel function. Diversion colitis is associated with worse function at 6 months after stoma closure,[49] and meta-analysis has demonstrated increased anastomotic stricture in diverted patients.[46] A large retrospective study demonstrated equivalent functional outcomes, however.[44] More rigorous data on the functional consequences of diversion are needed to elucidate this relationship.

Radiotherapy

Several large, multicenter randomized trials have found that radiotherapy (RT) is a highly significant risk factor for postoperative bowel dysfunction,[50–52] with more patients suffering from urgency, frequency, and dependence on antidiarrheal medications even 12 to 24 months after treatment.[50] The Dutch TME trial, using patient-reported instruments, demonstrated higher rates of fecal incontinence (62% vs 38%), higher frequency of bowel movements (3.7 vs 3.0 daily), and greater pad dependence even at 5 years postoperatively in patients randomized to preoperative RT.[53] Meta-analysis has shown a risk ratio of 1.67 for incontinence with neoadjuvant RT versus surgery alone as well as worsening of manometric anorectal function measurements.[52]

Timing of RT may also affect function. Results of the German Rectal Cancer Study Group trial indicate decreased gastrointestinal toxicity in preoperative RT compared with postoperative RT, with significantly less acute diarrhea (12% vs 18%) and less long-term gastrointestinal dysfunction (composite of diarrhea and small bowel obstruction; 9% vs 15%) in the preoperative RT group.[51]

RT causes significant bowel dysfunction, and the functional consequences of RT should be considered when planning treatment of rectal cancer. Data on function in patients treated with initial nonoperative management[54] remains to be seen. Studies such as the Alliance PROSPECT trial, which is evaluating the role of selective radiation, may provide important information on decreasing long-term sequelae of treatment while maintaining good oncologic outcomes.

Chemotherapy

There are few studies evaluating the long-term effects of modern neoadjuvant or adjuvant chemotherapy, but investigation of the consequences of combined chemoradiotherapy (CRT) have not shown differences in incontinence or frequency.[55–57] A randomized trial comparing RT to CRT and evaluating QOL is currently being conducted in Germany.[58] Adjuvant chemotherapy, such as oxaliplatin, although known to have neurotoxicity, has never been studied as an independent factor in bowel dysfunction. Although the current body of literature is limited, the impact of chemotherapy on long-term function is likely overshadowed by the effects of radiation when given in combination.

SEXUAL FUNCTION

Sexual function after treatment of colorectal cancer is less understood than bowel function but can have a profound effect on patients after treatment. Unlike the obligatory nature of bowel and urinary function, sexual function is discretionary and heavily influenced by individual social, psychological, and cultural factors, even under normal circumstances. Due to the contextual complexity and private nature of sexual function, it is a challenging factor to quantify. Furthermore, sexual dysfunction has different manifestations associated with gender, further obfuscating understanding by reducing analyzable sample sizes and preventing cross-gender comparison.

Lack of sexual activity cannot be used as a surrogate for sexual dysfunction. In addition to physiologic capability, sexual activity requires desire and opportunity, which are in turn subject to a patient's social and psychological state, partner status and partner's psychosociologic status, cultural influences, home environment, and other baseline characteristics. Patients diagnosed with cancer and their families undergo considerable psychological and social stressors that can affect sexual function. Measuring and accounting for these many variables is challenging, especially when the goal is to use concise instruments that can be administered repeatedly to a sufficiently large population.

Colon Cancer

Little is known about the effects of colon cancer on sexual function. Changes in sexual function in colon cancer patients are likely closely related to a patient's general health throughout treatment, and there are many significant contextual effects after diagnosis and during treatment. Few data exist, but a large population-based survey of colon cancer survivors demonstrated fewer male sexual problems and greater sexual enjoyment in chemotherapy recipients than in nonchemotherapy patients; the chemotherapy patients were significantly younger (mean age 66 vs 72 years),[59] although they also had more advanced disease. Although sexual function may be affected after treatment of colon cancer, a small cross-sectional study of women, comparing LAR patients treated with TME against postcolectomy patients, found that the colectomy patients scored better in all domains.[60] Likewise, a survey of male colorectal cancer survivors found rectal cancer the most predictive factor for impotence.[61] Nonetheless, sexual dysfunction has likely been under-reported in men undergoing sigmoid resection and should be further evaluated. Although the neurotoxicity of platinum-based chemotherapy may affect sexual function, this has not been reported. Sexual function in patients treated for colon cancer most likely closely mimics that of the general age-matched population over time. Additional research is required to define the effects of colon cancer on long-term sexual function.

Rectal Cancer

The burden of sexual dysfunction after rectal cancer therapy is considerable. A cross-sectional study of rectal cancer survivors found that 43% of sexually active men and 39% of sexually active women had sexual dysfunction,[62] findings corroborated by other studies.[63,64] In a separate prospective longitudinal study, the incidence of new sexual dysfunction in men was 66% at 3 months, improving in 14% by 6 months.[65] In a systematic review of the literature, 30% to 40% of patients reporting sexual activity preoperatively became inactive postoperatively.[66]

Nerve injury and scarring are hypothesized as significant factors in sexual dysfunction. In a prospective study of autonomic nerve sacrifice, ligation of the superior hypogastric plexus was associated with disorders of ejaculation, whereas ligation of the inferior hypogastric plexus was associated with impotence.[67] In female patients, such separation of functions remains more theoretic, but injury to sympathetic nerves is expected to reduce internal sensation, orgasm, and lubrication, whereas injury to parasympathetic nerves is expected to reduce labial engorgement, which may lead to dyspareunia. In addition to nerve injury, pelvic scarring, particularly in women, may also manifest symptomatically.

Patient Factors

Because sexual activity varies so much in the general population, it might be expected that patient-related variables that influence sexual activity have an impact on post-treatment sexual activity, potentially confounding analyses of post-treatment sexual dysfunction.

Age

Age has been shown to affect sexual activity in the general population. Despite a possible increase in sexual activity in the geriatric population with the increasing availability of pharmacologic aids, a reference sample published in 2007 found rates of sexual activity to decrease with age: from 73% to 53% to 26% in populations aged 57 to 64, 65 to 74, and 75 to 85 years, respectively.[66] Findings by Hendren and colleagues[62] support this result, documenting, by linear regression, a year-by-year odds ratio of 0.94 of continuing sexual activity with advancing age. Other studies have concurred, finding an independent association between age and poor sexual function postoperatively.[65,68] A study using a modified version of the European Organisation for Research and Treatment of Cancer (EORTC) instrument found that younger patients experienced higher levels of "personal strain" due to postoperative sexual dysfunction than older patients.[69] Younger patients are more likely to be sexually active and also more likely to suffer due to postsurgical impairment of their sexual function. These considerations are important when comparing studies of sexual function after cancer treatment and also during patient counseling and treatment planning.

Gender

Assessing the effects of gender on post-treatment dysfunction is particularly challenging. There may be an elevated risk of nerve damage during dissection in the narrow male pelvis,[70] but because of differences in the details and assessment instruments of male and female dysfunction, direct comparison has not been effective. Postoperative dysfunction has been studied more extensively in men, and evidence in women has been particularly poor for several reasons, including issues in measurement (the older EORTC QLQ-CR38 module systematically excludes information from sexually inactive women), lower response rates to surveys of sexual function among women, and the discrete nature of male dysfunction.[66] More study of female sexual dysfunction, as well as an instrument that allows comparison with men, is needed to determine if there is a gender bias in post-treatment dysfunction.

Preoperative function

Preoperative sexual activity and function can be expected to be major determinants of postoperative dysfunction, but few studies have adequately measured preoperative function or assessed the relationship. Patients who are inactive preoperatively rarely become active postoperatively; in a bi-gender sample, Hendren and colleagues[62] found that preoperative activity was the strongest predictor of postoperative activity, with an odds ratio of 37.8, underscoring the importance of its assessment. More recently, others have also found that preoperative dysfunction predicts dysfunction at 3 and 6 months postoperatively.[65] To adequately understand the effects of treatment, the preoperative sexual activity and functionality of patients must be considered.

Tumor Factors

Tumor level

Tumor height determines depth and difficulty of dissection and, thereby, potentially affects postoperative sexual function. In a retrospective of laparoscopic TME (84% LAR and 16% APR), logistic regression identified male patients with tumors greater than 7 cm from the anal verge as much more likely to be capable of erection compared with those with lower tumors, with an odds ratio of 45.5.[71] Anterior or anterolateral tumors in men are likely to affect sexual function more than posterior tumors because of the position of the hypogastric nerves at the level of the prostate.

Tumor stage

Few data exist on the effect of tumor stage on sexual function. In a retrospective analysis,[71] stage was not found to predict sexual function. It could be hypothesized that T4 tumors invading beyond the mesorectal sheath require wider resections, and tumors penetrating the thin anterior mesorectum pose the greatest threat to sexual function, with hypogastric neurovascular bundles coursing through the adjacent Denonvilliers fascia. Although tumor stage was not specified, Hendren and colleagues[72] reported on the sexual function of a cohort of women who underwent en bloc proctectomy with partial or complete vaginectomy. Rates of sexual activity decreased from 48% to 30%, and 39% of patients reported being incapable of sexual activity due to insufficient vaginal capacity, dyspareunia, or chronic perineal wounds. Advanced tumors requiring multivisceral resections place patients at considerable risk for sexual dysfunction. Further research in this area is necessary.

Treatment Factors

Minimally invasive technique

Existing data on minimally invasive TME are mixed. Early outcomes from the multicenter randomized CLASICC trial suggest greater sexual dysfunction after laparoscopic surgery, with 41% incidence of severely worsened function compared with 26% in the open surgery group.[73] Similarly, in a follow-up of another randomized trial, survivors who were sexually active preoperatively were significantly more likely to be impotent or sexually impaired if they had undergone laparoscopic (40.0%) compared with open surgery (13.6%).[64] Newer data have reached opposing conclusions, however, although from non-randomized studies. Men who underwent laparoscopy demonstrated less dysfunction and better satisfaction at 12 to 18 months[74] and lower rates of postoperative impotence (1/18 patients vs 6/17) compared with men who underwent open procedures[75]; sexually active women who underwent laparoscopic surgery were also less likely to have reduced function postoperatively (1/14 patients) compared with the open group (5/10 patients).[75] The robotic approach, which is increasingly being used to perform TME, may have benefits over laparoscopic surgery. A recent prospective study comparing laparoscopic and robotic TME found both groups had a deterioration of sexual function at 1 month postoperatively; however, most patients in the robotic group returned to baseline function by 6 months postoperatively, whereas most patients in the laparoscopic group required 12 months to recover function.[76] Patient-reported outcomes from the multicenter randomized COLOR II and ACOSOG Z6051 trials may provide further insight.

TME and non-TME approaches

Prior to the advent of TME, sexual dysfunction after rectal cancer surgery was extremely pervasive, as high as 70% to 100%[77,78]; some surgeons considered sexual dysfunction a marker of oncologically adequate resection.[66] TME has resulted in significant improvement in sexual function.

Two other, nonstandard TME approaches have reported data on sexual function. ELND increases the risk to autonomic nerves and has been shown a strong predictor of sexual dysfunction postoperatively,[79] with a decrease in sexual activity from 90% to 50% and in ejaculation from 70% to 10%, when ELND was added to TME.[80] A prospective study from Japan compared male patients undergoing standard TME to patients undergoing TME + ELND, further stratifying them by extent of pelvic nerve preservation, and found that patients in the standard TME group were able to maintain intercourse and nocturnal rigidity at a rate of 95% versus 56%, 45%, and 0% for TME + ELND in patients with bilateral, unilateral, and no nerve preservation, respectively.[81]

Given that local excision of tumors does not impact nerve plexi, transanal techniques could be expected to produce much better sexual outcomes. The literature on this subject is scant, but one prospective study on TEM patients found no change in any sexual item of the EORTC-CR38 when comparing presurgery to 3, 6, and 12 months postsurgery,[24] suggesting that local excision preserves sexual function very well.

LAR versus APR

Several studies comparing LAR to APR have consistently found APR associated with worse sexual function.[66,82,83] APR may be associated with more pain from pelvic and perineal scarring and sensory changes as well as possible avulsion of the sphlanchnic nerves from the sacral roots.[70] A meta-analysis of QOL after the two procedures found APR is significantly associated with lower sexual function scores and more male sexual problems.[84] A study of female patients also found decreased activity and a 5.8-fold increase in incidence of dyspareunia with APR.[68] In the bigender cross-sectional study by Hendren and colleagues,[62] patients who underwent LAR had a much higher likelihood (OR 3.5) of being sexually active compared with those who underwent APR. Even for tumors of equal height,[85] function seems worse after APR compared with LAR. There are no studies comparing the sexual function of patients undergoing a hand-sewn coloanal anastomosis to patients undergoing APR. At present, the literature suggests that sexual function is better after LAR than APR.

Ostomy

Separating the impact of an ostomy from the other aspects of APR is difficult, with a dearth of literature to isolate the effects of either colostomy or diverting ileostomy on sexual function. Ostomies seem to have a unique impact on QOL, particularly with respect to body image and feelings of embarrassment that may affect sexual interest or enjoyment in a patient or partner. Thus, ostomies have the potential to profoundly affect sexual function.

Although the true impact of a stoma remains confounded by the consequences of extensive pelvic dissection, there is evidence that sexual function is diminished by more than nerve injury alone. One study reported no significant difference in QOL between patients with and without a stoma but found that stoma patients reported a nonsignificantly lower mean sexual enjoyment (17 vs 67 out of 100) and significantly worse body image.[86] Another found that stoma-related problems were significantly associated with worse QOL, reporting a nonsignificantly lower median score for overall male sexual dysfunction in ostomy patients versus nonstomates (66 and 83, respectively).[87] Other studies have corroborated simultaneous diminishment of sexual and social functions.[88] Issues surrounding body image are prevalent among patients with a stoma.

Radiotherapy

RT is an important component of therapy for many patients with rectal cancer, but it significantly affects postoperative sexual function. RT increases the likelihood that patients describe their sexual life as worsened after treatment by a factor of 5.6.[62] The multicenter Dutch trial, randomizing patients to preoperative RT versus surgery alone, demonstrates significantly worsened overall sexual function in both men and women after neoadjuvant RT, specifically noting greater erectile and ejaculatory dysfunction that continued to deteriorate over time.[89] A population-based Norwegian follow-up of survivors demonstrated significantly diminished erection, orgasm, intercourse, and overall sexual satisfaction, reporting an increase in moderate-to-severe erectile dysfunction by a factor of 7.3 when RT was used. A recent meta-analysis reported significantly worse male sexual function after RT but did not demonstrate clear evidence of worsening of female sexual function.[52] Radiation, however, is known to potentially cause vaginal changes, including shortening, atrophy, fibrosis, adhesions, dryness, dyspareunia, and premature ovarian failure.[70] The effects of timing of RT on sexual function have not been studied, but a retrospective analysis found that both neoadjuvant and adjuvant CRT were predictive of male sexual dysfunction.[71] Pelvic RT has detrimental effects on sexual function.

Chemotherapy

Chemotherapy, especially platinum-based treatment, has a hypothetical risk of causing or exacerbating sexual dysfunction. Further research is needed, but the current literature suggests that chemotherapy does not negatively affect sexual function.

URINARY FUNCTION

The third domain of post-treatment dysfunction after rectal cancer therapy is urinary dysfunction.

Colon Cancer

Urinary dysfunction after colorectal cancer treatment results from nerve damage and inflammation in the pelvis after pelvic dissection or radiation. Colon cancer patients are relatively spared these effects; in general, urinary symptoms are transient and result from urinary tract infections or underlying prostatic hypertrophy.

Rectal Cancer

After rectal cancer treatment, the burden of postoperative urinary dysfunction is high. The multicenter Dutch TME trial reported that, among patients who were continent preoperatively, new urinary incontinence occurred at rates of 27% at 5 years postsurgery (38% overall, in a population with 28% preoperative incontinence) and new difficulty emptying occurred at rates of 19.9% (30.6% overall, in a population with 35.0% preoperative difficulty emptying).[90] In nonrandomized trials, urinary dysfunction is common after treatment, with postproctectomy urinary dysfunction rates reportedly between 30% and 70%.[91]

Manifestations of postoperative urinary dysfunction range from difficulty retaining urine to difficulty emptying the bladder, and the multiple causes of unintentional spillage. Irritative symptomatology, or storage dysfunction, results from detrusor muscle instability and sympathetic impairment, believed to result from injury to the superior hypogastric plexus or hypogastric nerves. Premature contraction and reduced bladder capacity manifest as intense urinary urge, frequency, nocturia, and possible urge incontinence. Obstructive symptomatology, or voiding dysfunction, results from impairment of detrusor contraction or sphincter/ureteral relaxation after parasympathetic injury to the inferior hypogastric plexus and manifests as difficulty emptying the bladder, painful or bothersome retention, and possible overflow incontinence. Additionally, stress incontinence can occur due to alteration of pelvic anatomic relations after surgical dissection, causing insufficient structural support to urovesicular organs. In contrast to sexual dysfunction, urinary dysfunction is usually more transient. Temporary dysfunction, due to perivesicular inflammation, detrusor hypoactivity, or diminished bladder sensation, is common in the early postoperative period, often resolving within 3 and 6 months with healing and nerve regeneration. Dysfunction persisting at 1 year postoperatively is usually permanent.[70]

Patient Factors

Age

Prevalence of urinary dysfunction increases in the elderly; likewise, increasing age independently associates with greater dysfunction after treatment of rectal cancer. EORTC micturition scores are worse in patients over 80 years of age compared with those under 70[10] and postoperative nocturia occurs more frequently in females over age 65, by a factor of 2.1 after multivariate adjustment for preoperative function.[68] Increasing urinary dysfunction associated with age can impede the study of long-term outcomes, because cancer patients are often elderly at time of surgery and have a high incidence of developing or worsening age-related urinary dysfunction in the follow-up period.

Gender

Profiles of urinary dysfunction differ by gender in the general population, with greater incontinence in women and greater obstructive dysfunction in men. Gender is also a strong predictor of post-treatment incontinence after rectal cancer, occurring in women with an odds ratio of 2.7.[90] Multiple gender-specific factors predispose women to incontinence, including childbirth and history of hysterectomy, which result in worsened urinary dysfunction after proctectomy.[92] Postmenopausal status is believed to play a role in female incontinence, because lack of estrogen stimulation modulates the pelvic floor muscles to laxity[90]; menopausal status should be accounted for in the study of female urinary dysfunction. In general, female gender may predispose patients to greater incontinence after rectal cancer therapy.

Preoperative function
As might be expected, preoperative urinary dysfunction is a strong predictor of post-treatment dysfunction. In the Dutch TME trial, preoperative incontinence was independently associated with post-treatment incontinence (OR 2.75), and preoperative emptying difficulty was independently associated with emptying difficulty postoperatively (OR 2.94).[90]

Tumor Factors

Tumor level
Tumor level has often been confounded by choice of APR. As discussed later, APR and, therefore, lower tumors are significantly correlated with postoperative urinary dysfunction. This may be because injury to the muscles of the pelvic floor causes weakening of the urinary sphincter.[90]

Tumor stage
In a retrospective study, Morino and colleagues[71] found that stage III patients were more likely to suffer postoperative urinary dysfunction than patients with earlier stage disease; however, this small study did not account for preoperative status or confounding by radiotherapy, which was administered to late stage patients only. Tumors on the anterior or anterolateral walls of the rectum pose the greatest threat to urinary function—especially T4 tumors, because there is potential for injury to the hypogastric nerves that run between layers of Denonvilliers fascia, anterolateral to the rectum, and posterolateral to the prostate and seminal vesicles.[93]

Treatment Factors

Open versus minimally invasive technique
Minimally invasive surgical techniques may potentially affect the quality of dissection in TME, because they increase visualization and magnification and afford the use of very fine instruments but also decrease tactile feedback and may produce inferior retraction. Laparoscopic dissection in the anterolateral plane, where the hypogastric nerves travel, is particularly difficult.[70] When evaluated in the CLASICC trial, no difference in urinary dysfunction was seen in laparoscopic versus open groups.[73] Although several small observational studies have been conducted, the multicenter randomized COLOR II and ACOSOG Z6051 trials may provide additional insight.

TME and non-TME approaches
Proper TME technique is critically important to the preservation of urinary function. Although bladder dysfunction remains prevalent, adoption of TME technique over wide excision has improved rates of urinary problems, from 50% to 60% to 20% to 30%.[78] This advantage is attributed to improved preservation of the hypogastric nerves; injury to pelvic autonomic nerves was reported in 25% of cases in the Dutch TME trial, which found this a significant predictor of postoperative emptying difficulty (OR 2.82).[70] Even single-side nerve preservation of the inferior hypogastric plexus may

be sufficient to prevent incontinence.[90] Use of nerve-sparing TME technique has reportedly reduced minor incontinence to 19%, major incontinence to 0%, and irritative/frequency problems to 22% in long-term follow-up between 1 and 2 years postsurgery.[67]

ELND is associated with increased urinary dysfunction. Lymph node dissection may lead to devascularization or even inadvertent ligation of pelvic autonomic nerves.[94] In a prospective study examining ELND and nerve preservation in TME patients, rates of urinary retention were low without ELND (4%) but increased to 27% with ELND even when bilateral pelvic plexi were preserved; urinary retention rates increased further, to 77% and 100% with unilateral sparing or no sparing, respectively.[81]

Given that local excision of tumors does not impact nerve plexi, transanal techniques could be expected to result in improved urinary outcomes. The literature on the subject is scant, but one prospective study following TEM patients found no change in any urinary item of the EORTC-CR38 from before surgery to 3, 6, and 12 months after surgery,[24] suggesting that local excision preserves urinary function well. Further research is needed, but initial reports suggest that TEM has less impact on urinary function than more invasive surgical techniques.

LAR versus APR

APR has been associated with significantly increased postoperative urinary dysfunction. Potential physiologic mechanisms include injury to the innervation of the levator ani muscles,[90] subsequently causing sphincteric laxity, or posterior sagging of the bladder into the empty pelvis, causing pelvic floor deformity. Increased urinary dysfunction after APR compared with LAR has been demonstrated in multiple studies,[80,92] and APR in women is specifically correlated with urinary retention (OR 11.7), poor stream (OR 5.6), and incontinence (OR 2.4).[68] APR produces significant urinary morbidity.

Radiotherapy

RT has been known to cause significant urinary dysfunction in the treatment of prostate cancer, causing fibrosis of the bladder and urinary sphincters, with functional consequences.[70] An early randomized trial found that preoperative RT was associated with urinary incontinence (45% in the RT group vs 27% for surgery alone).[95] In the larger, randomized Dutch TME trial, however, RT was not independently associated with urinary dysfunction.[90] The effects of RT on urinary dysfunction in rectal cancer remain unclear.

Chemotherapy

Chemotherapy, especially platinum-based treatments, pose a hypothetical risk of causing or exacerbating urinary dysfunction via neurotoxicity to the pelvic autonomic nerves, which may already be in jeopardy after dissection. Current literature does not suggest that chemotherapy is related to postoperative urinary dysfunction, but further research is needed.

FUTURE DIRECTIONS
Improving Measurement

Bowel function measurement

Although bowel dysfunction is evident in colorectal cancer patients, understanding the extent of the problem is challenging. Cohorts have been largely retrospective, and assessment of function is varied, making the data difficult to assimilate.[34] Many studies have used older, symptom-specific scales developed to measure individual symptoms, including the Wexner (Cleveland Clinic) Incontinence Score, the Fecal

Incontinence Severity Index, and other scales.[96] These scales are too limited in scope to assess the various manifestations of bowel dysfunction after rectal cancer and focus on specific issues, such as continence. Although bowel function items exist on most QOL measures, their discriminatory power has been questioned.[97]

Recently, better-tailored instruments have been developed to improve understanding of function and QOL after colorectal cancer treatments. These include the Memorial Sloan-Kettering Cancer Center Bowel Function Instrument[8] and the shorter Low Anterior Resection Syndrome score, specifically designed and validated as having discriminatory power capable of measuring dysfunction after sphincter-preserving surgery for rectal cancer using psychometric methodology.[98] Expanding the use of comprehensive, validated questionnaires should lead to more rigorous assessment of bowel function and improve the generalizability of knowledge within the field.

Sexual function measurement

Measurement of sexual function is limited compared with other outcomes and is studied without sufficient rigor. Assessment of preoperative activity and function, desire, opportunity, and psychiatric state are all important components. Poor measurement has limited understanding of the scope and features of post-treatment sexual dysfunction.

There is potential for better measurement of sexual function going forward. Although the EORTC QLQ-CR38[66] had 5 items on sexual function, it excluded information from sexually inactive women. It has recently been updated, shortened, and validated as the QLQ-CR29[99] and may provide some ability to do cross-gender comparisons. Alternatively, more detailed, gender-specific, patient-reported sexual function instruments have also been used: the Female Sexual Function Index, and the International Index of Erectile Function. These instruments have set a standard for detail and rigor in measuring assessment and treatment of sexual dysfunction, but further research with these instruments is necessary to establish norms in rectal cancer patients.

Urinary function measurement

Much like other domains of dysfunction after rectal cancer treatment, the understanding of post-treatment urinary dysfunction has been hampered by inconsistency in definitions and measurement methodologies. The range of assessment tools used to measure urinary dysfunction is wider still than that of bowel or sexual function instruments, encompassing discrete clinical endpoints, such as catheter use, urodynamic physiologic measures, and a variety of nonvalidated patient-reported survey instruments. Lack of standardization significantly hampers cross-study comparisons.

One of the most widely used instruments has been the EORTC QLQ-CR38 module, which contains 1 micturition subscale. Its replacement, the validated QLQ-CR29, has 4 items regarding urinary function: daytime and nighttime frequency, incontinence, and dysuria. Another frequently used scale is the International Prostate Symptom Score. Designed for the male population and used widely by urologists, it covers a broader range of symptoms, ties symptoms to QOL, and can be used in female patients. Development of a standardized method of assessment would improve interpretability and comparability of research results. Consensus and widespread utilization of a single standard patient-reported instrument is needed to further the study of postoperative urinary dysfunction.

Injury Prevention

Although all investigators advocate sharp mesorectal dissection and identification of nerves, some also advocate intraoperative nerve stimulation and monitoring. A small case-controlled study found significantly less incontinence in patients after TME with intraoperative nerve monitoring (IONM) compared with TME without IONM (6.7% vs 40%).[100] Additional studies of IONM have found that identification of parasympathetic nerves was highly correlated with improvement in urologic outcomes, reducing early urinary dysfunction to 26.7% and long-term urinary dysfunction to 18%,[101] with 95% normal sexual function in patients with nerves deemed intact at time of surgery.[102] A prospective assessment of the test attributes of intraoperative monitoring found erectile dysfunction in 26.7% of patients, with a specificity of 89% and accuracy of 77% for predicting normal sexual function if nerves had been identified.[101] These results are provocative and suggest that wider use of IONM has the potential to help prevent inadvertent nerve injuries. IONM increases the length and cost of surgery, however, and has not yet been widely adopted. IONM should be tested in a larger, blinded randomized trial to further establish its efficacy.

Changing the treatment paradigm may also result in improvement in bowel, sexual, and bladder dysfunction. For instance, in the setting of low rectal tumors, nonoperative management of patients who have had a clinical complete response to CRT with or without chemotherapy has potential promise, although more prospective data are required. Alternatively, for midrectal tumors, selective radiation may result in equivalent oncologic outcomes and better functional results in all domains. Results of the Alliance for Clinical Trials in Oncology PROSPECT trial will provide important information about selective radiation.

Treating Dysfunction

Treating bowel dysfunction

Management of bowel dysfunction commonly includes symptom-driven dietary adjustments and adjustments in medication. The role of physical therapy and biofeedback for treating incontinence after rectal surgery has been reported only in small series, with limited outcomes. Anal sphincter training significantly decreases frequency and improves depression and perceived QOL.[103] Manipulation of bowel flora via antibiotics has been studied at the authors' institution, and results are pending.

Use of sacral neuromodulation in postcancer bowel dysfunction is another area of interesting therapeutic potential. Studies of incontinent patients demonstrate that, at 4 to 5 years postimplant, incontinent episodes decreased from 9.4 to 1.9 per week,[104] self-reported function and well-being significantly improved, and 73% of patients reported satisfaction.[105] Sacral neuromodulation for patients with posttreatment bowel dysfunction has been evaluated in a small series and demonstrated dramatic improvement, reducing incontinence episodes by 60% (from 20 to 8 times weekly) and reducing soiling, urgency, and fragmentation in two-thirds of patients, significantly improving QOL.[106] Although larger, comparative studies are needed, sacral neuromodulation may prove an excellent option for reducing postoperative dysfunction.

Treating sexual dysfunction

Recovery of sexual function after significant injury sustained during treatment is problematic. Function can continue to worsen between 3 and 12 months postprocedure,[107] and any spontaneous recovery tends to be slow and incomplete.[108]

Various methods have been used to treat postoperative sexual dysfunction. In men, the typical first-line treatment is oral sildenafil, which was evaluated in a randomized, double-blind, placebo-controlled trial with excellent results. At a median 5.6 years postoperatively, 79% receiving sildenafil reported improvement in erectile function, compared with only 3% of patients receiving placebo.[109] Data from subsequent prospective studies have been mixed, with some studies reporting similarly excellent results[79]; other studies show no success with oral sildenafil but demonstrate some improvement, sufficient for intercourse, with intracavernous injection therapy.[110] Other treatment options not studied in rectal cancer patients, but with therapeutic potential, include intraurethral prostaglandin E, vacuum systems, implantable prosthetics,[111] or nerve interposition grafts.[70] Psychological interventions have been studied as well at the authors' institution.

There has been no systematic investigation of treatments of female sexual dysfunction. Commonly recommended therapies include vaginal lubricants or topical estrogens for dryness and vaginal dilators and pelvic floor muscle exercises for stenosis, which may be used prophylactically.[111] Hyperbaric oxygen therapy has also been suggested for chronic perineal injuries.[70] Sexual health education coupled with psychosexual counseling in women with sexual dysfunction after rectal cancer may also provide some benefit. Significant work can be done in this area to improve outcomes in women.

Treating urinary dysfunction

Several treatments have been used for urinary dysfunction after rectal cancer surgery. Patients with acute urinary retention are often discharged on tamsulosin and/or with an indwelling Foley catheter, these measures may be discontinued as postoperative pelvic inflammation subsides. Patients with urge incontinence or urinary frequency may benefit from oxybutynin. Patients with stress incontinence may respond well to pelvic floor muscular exercises to improve strength and control of the urethral sphincter, although the success of such techniques may be limited if the pelvic floor is significantly denervated.[70] Sacral nerve stimulation was first developed to manage urinary incontinence, and has become a major treatment alternative in this domain.[112,113] Chronic indwelling or suprapubic catheterization can be used to treat dysfunction when other measures fail, although catheterization carries the morbidity of recurrent and potentially life-threatening urinary tract infections. Patients with persistent urinary dysfunction should be referred to a urologist for evaluation.

SUMMARY

With significant improvements in survival after colorectal cancer, functional outcomes of treatment are an increasing focus of both patients and practitioners. Although there is a relative paucity of literature, colon cancer treatment seems to have an effect on long-term function. In comparison with rectal cancer patients, however, colon cancer patients experience significantly fewer long-term functional alterations.

The current body of literature is difficult to assimilate. Many studies are retrospective, omit important clinical details, or use nonvalidated measurement tools. Given the multitude of factors that affect function, large studies are required to obtain meaningful data. Understanding the interplay between bowel, sexual, and bladder function and its impact on QOL will help improve treatment. Although there is some evidence that patients adapt to functional changes or presence of an ostomy over time,[97] it is important to understand the psychological and cognitive processes that occur during this adaptation.

Although the literature is incomplete, it is possible to provide some information to patients about their expected postoperative function. Several factors can be used to identify patients who are likely to experience more dysfunction. Preoperative bowel, sexual, and bladder function should be assessed. Although older age may be associated with worse function, younger patients seem to experience greater distress. Tumor factors have an impact on outcomes, with low tumors leading to worse functional outcomes. Tumor stage and location remain important areas for further study. The impact of treatment factors must also be considered. Data regarding the effects of minimally invasive surgery on function will be available after sufficient follow-up of the ACOSOG Z6051 trial. APR and ELND cause sexual and urinary dysfunction associated with nerve injury. Transanal local excision seems to conserve function in all domains. Pouch reconstruction, especially the J pouch, restores bowel function. Ostomy creation reduces sexual function, likely due to psychosocial factors. RT worsens both bowel and sexual function.

Ideally, function could be preserved after treatment of rectal cancer. In small series, IONM to limit injury seems to improve long-term outcomes, but this has not been thoroughly studied or widely adopted. Even with perfect surgical technique, however, some patients will probably still experience dysfunction. Perhaps the most effective method of improving functional outcomes will be in changing treatment paradigms to limit injury, as proposed by the Alliance PROSPECT selective radiation trial, and/or the development of a nonoperative management protocol in complete responders.

Treatment options for dysfunction after rectal cancer therapy are perhaps most lacking, and high-quality research is needed. Biofeedback and pelvic floor physical therapeutics, manipulation of bowel flora, psychosocial and pharmacologic interventions for sexual dysfunction, nerve grafts, and, especially, sacral nerve stimulation, show promise and should be investigated further. In addition, providing patients with appropriate psychological support as well as psychosocial interventions may also improve their ability to adapt to these significant post-treatment changes.

Impressive improvement in oncologic outcomes has been achieved in colorectal cancer. Given this, the importance of functional outcomes must be emphasized so that patients may enjoy their extended survival. Much remains to be done to improve function, and, as with any new treatment paradigm, function as an outcome must be measured and optimized.

REFERENCES

1. Nikoletti S, Young J, Levitt M, et al. Bowel problems, self-care practices, and information needs of colorectal cancer survivors at 6 to 24 months after sphincter-saving surgery. Cancer Nurs 2008;31(5):389–98.
2. Ohigashi S, Hoshino Y, Ohde S, et al. Functional outcome, quality of life, and efficacy of probiotics in postoperative patients with colorectal cancer. Surg Today 2011;41(9):1200–6.
3. Sato K, Inomata M, Kakisako K, et al. Surgical technique influences bowel function after low anterior resection and sigmoid colectomy. Hepatogastroenterology 2003;50(53):1381–4.
4. Ricciardi R, Virnig BA, Madoff RD, et al. The status of radical proctectomy and sphincter-sparing surgery in the United States. Dis Colon Rectum 2007;50(8):1119–27 [discussion: 1126–7].
5. Temple LK, Romanus D, Niland J, et al. Factors associated with sphincter-preserving surgery for rectal cancer at national comprehensive cancer network centers. Ann Surg 2009;250(2):260–7.
6. Weiser MR, Quah HM, Shia J, et al. Sphincter preservation in low rectal cancer is facilitated by preoperative chemoradiation and intersphincteric dissection. Ann Surg 2009;249(2):236–42.
7. Ziv Y, Gimelfarb Y, Igov I. Post anterior rectal resection syndrome—a retrospective multicentre study. Colorectal Dis 2013;15(6):e317–22.

8. Temple LK, Bacik J, Savatta SG, et al. The development of a validated instrument to evaluate bowel function after sphincter-preserving surgery for rectal cancer. Dis Colon Rectum 2005;48(7):1353–65.

9. Dehni N, Schlegel D, Tiret E, et al. Effects of aging on the functional outcome of coloanal anastomosis with colonic J-pouch. Am J Surg 1998;175(3):209–12.

10. Mastracci TM, Hendren S, O'Connor B, et al. The impact of surgery for colorectal cancer on quality of life and functional status in the elderly. Dis Colon Rectum 2006;49(12):1878–84.

11. Rasmussen OO, Petersen IK, Christiansen J. Anorectal function following low anterior resection. Colorectal Dis 2003;5(3):258–61.

12. Theodoropoulos GE, Papanikolaou IG, Karantanos T, et al. Post-colectomy assessment of gastrointestinal function: a prospective study on colorectal cancer patients. Tech Coloproctol 2013;17(5):525–36.

13. Zutshi M, Hull T, Shedda S, et al. Gender differences in mortality, quality of life and function after restorative procedures for rectal cancer. Colorectal Dis 2013; 15(1):66–73.

14. Denost Q, Laurent C, Capdepont M, et al. Risk factors for fecal incontinence after intersphincteric resection for rectal cancer. Dis Colon Rectum 2011;54(8): 963–8.

15. Bretagnol F, Troubat H, Laurent C, et al. Long-term functional results after sphincter-saving resection for rectal cancer. Gastroenterol Clin Biol 2004; 28(2):155–9.

16. Ho YH. Techniques for restoring bowel continuity and function after rectal cancer surgery. World J Gastroenterol 2006;12(39):6252–60.

17. Matzel KE, Stadelmaier U, Muehldorfer S, et al. Continence after colorectal reconstruction following resection: impact of level of anastomosis. Int J Colorectal Dis 1997;12(2):82–7.

18. Amin AI, Hallbook O, Lee AJ, et al. A 5-cm colonic J pouch colo-anal reconstruction following anterior resection for low rectal cancer results in acceptable evacuation and continence in the long term. Colorectal Dis 2003;5(1):33–7.

19. Bretagnol F, Rullier E, Laurent C, et al. Comparison of functional results and quality of life between intersphincteric resection and conventional coloanal anastomosis for low rectal cancer. Dis Colon Rectum 2004;47(6):832–8.

20. Martin ST, Heneghan HM, Winter DC. Systematic review of outcomes after intersphincteric resection for low rectal cancer. Br J Surg 2012;99(5): 603–12.

21. Andersson J, Angenete E, Gellerstedt M, et al. Health-related quality of life after laparoscopic and open surgery for rectal cancer in a randomized trial. Br J Surg 2013;100(7):941–9.

22. Matsuoka H, Masaki T, Sugiyama M, et al. Impact of lateral pelvic lymph node dissection on evacuatory and urinary functions following low anterior resection for advanced rectal carcinoma. Langenbecks Arch Surg 2005;390(6):517–22.

23. Fenech DS, Takahashi T, Liu M, et al. Function and quality of life after transanal excision of rectal polyps and cancers. Dis Colon Rectum 2007;50(5): 598–603.

24. Allaix ME, Rebecchi F, Giaccone C, et al. Long-term functional results and quality of life after transanal endoscopic microsurgery. Br J Surg 2011;98(11): 1635–43.

25. Jiang JK, Lin JK. Does anastomotic method affect functional outcome of low anterior resection for rectal carcinoma? Zhonghua Yi Xue Za Zhi (Taipei) 1997;60(5):252–8.

26. Laurent A, Parc Y, McNamara D, et al. Colonic J-pouch-anal anastomosis for rectal cancer: a prospective, randomized study comparing handsewn vs. stapled anastomosis. Dis Colon Rectum 2005;48(4):729–34.
27. Nesbakken A, Nygaard K, Lunde OC. Mesorectal excision for rectal cancer: functional outcome after low anterior resection and colorectal anastomosis without a reservoir. Colorectal Dis 2002;4(3):172–6.
28. Benoist S, Panis Y, Boleslawski E, et al. Functional outcome after coloanal versus low colorectal anastomosis for rectal carcinoma. J Am Coll Surg 1997; 185(2):114–9.
29. Chew SB, Tindal DS. Colonic J-pouch as a neorectum: functional assessment. Aust N Z J Surg 1997;67(9):607–10.
30. Dehni N, Tiret E, Singland JD, et al. Long-term functional outcome after low anterior resection: comparison of low colorectal anastomosis and colonic J-pouch-anal anastomosis. Dis Colon Rectum 1998;41(7):817–22 [discussion: 822–3].
31. Lin JK, Wang HS, Yang SH, et al. Comparison between straight and J-pouch coloanal anastomoses in surgery for rectal cancer. Surg Today 2002;32(6):487–92.
32. Doeksen A, Bakx R, Vincent A, et al. J-pouch vs side-to-end coloanal anastomosis after preoperative radiotherapy and total mesorectal excision for rectal cancer: a multicentre randomized trial. Colorectal Dis 2012;14(6):705–13.
33. Hida J, Yoshifuji T, Okuno K, et al. Long-term functional outcome of colonic J-pouch reconstruction after low anterior resection for rectal cancer. Surg Today 2006;36(5):441–9.
34. Brown CJ, Fenech DS, McLeod RS. Reconstructive techniques after rectal resection for rectal cancer. Cochrane Database Syst Rev 2008;(2):CD006040.
35. Lazorthes F, Gamagami R, Chiotasso P, et al. Prospective, randomized study comparing clinical results between small and large colonic J-pouch following coloanal anastomosis. Dis Colon Rectum 1997;40(12):1409–13.
36. Heah SM, Seow-Choen F, Eu KW, et al. Prospective, randomized trial comparing sigmoid vs. descending colonic J-pouch after total rectal excision. Dis Colon Rectum 2002;45(3):322–8.
37. Ho YH, Brown S, Heah SM, et al. Comparison of J-pouch and coloplasty pouch for low rectal cancers: a randomized, controlled trial investigating functional results and comparative anastomotic leak rates. Ann Surg 2002;236(1):49–55.
38. Furst A, Suttner S, Agha A, et al. Colonic J-pouch vs. coloplasty following resection of distal rectal cancer: early results of a prospective, randomized, pilot study. Dis Colon Rectum 2003;46(9):1161–6.
39. Biondo S, Frago R, Codina Cazador A, et al. Long-term functional results from a randomized clinical study of transverse coloplasty compared with colon J-pouch after low anterior resection for rectal cancer. Surgery 2013;153(3): 383–92.
40. Fazio VW, Zutshi M, Remzi FH, et al. A randomized multicenter trial to compare long-term functional outcome, quality of life, and complications of surgical procedures for low rectal cancers. Ann Surg 2007;246(3):481–8 [discussion: 488–90].
41. Zhang YC, Jin XD, Zhang YT, et al. Better functional outcome provided by short-armed sigmoid colon-rectal side-to-end anastomosis after laparoscopic low anterior resection: a match-paired retrospective study from China. Int J Colorectal Dis 2012;27(4):535–41.
42. Jiang JK, Yang SH, Lin JK. Transabdominal anastomosis after low anterior resection: A prospective, randomized, controlled trial comparing long-term results between side-to-end anastomosis and colonic J-pouch. Dis Colon Rectum 2005;48(11):2100–8 [discussion: 2108–10].

43. Machado M, Nygren J, Goldman S, et al. Similar outcome after colonic pouch and side-to-end anastomosis in low anterior resection for rectal cancer: a prospective randomized trial. Ann Surg 2003;238(2):214–20.

44. Remzi FH, Fazio VW, Gorgun E, et al. The outcome after restorative proctocolectomy with or without defunctioning ileostomy. Dis Colon Rectum 2006;49(4): 470–7.

45. Tan WS, Tang CL, Shi L, et al. Meta-analysis of defunctioning stomas in low anterior resection for rectal cancer. Br J Surg 2009;96(5):462–72.

46. Weston-Petrides GK, Lovegrove RE, Tilney HS, et al. Comparison of outcomes after restorative proctocolectomy with or without defunctioning ileostomy. Arch Surg 2008;143(4):406–12.

47. Montedori A, Cirocchi R, Farinella E, et al. Covering ileo- or colostomy in anterior resection for rectal carcinoma. Cochrane Database Syst Rev 2010;(5):CD006878.

48. Huser N, Michalski CW, Erkan M, et al. Systematic review and meta-analysis of the role of defunctioning stoma in low rectal cancer surgery. Ann Surg 2008; 248(1):52–60.

49. Son DN, Choi DJ, Woo SU, et al. Relationship between diversion colitis and quality of life in rectal cancer. World J Gastroenterol 2013;19(4):542–9.

50. Parc Y, Zutshi M, Zalinski S, et al. Preoperative radiotherapy is associated with worse functional results after coloanal anastomosis for rectal cancer. Dis Colon Rectum 2009;52(12):2004–14.

51. Sauer R, Becker H, Hohenberger W, et al. Preoperative versus postoperative chemoradiotherapy for rectal cancer. N Engl J Med 2004;351(17):1731–40.

52. Loos M, Quentmeier P, Schuster T, et al. Effect of preoperative radio(chemo) therapy on long-term functional outcome in rectal cancer patients: a systematic review and meta-analysis. Ann Surg Oncol 2013;20(6):1816–28.

53. Lange MM, den Dulk M, Bossema ER, et al. Risk factors for faecal incontinence after rectal cancer treatment. Br J Surg 2007;94(10):1278–84.

54. Smith JD, Ruby JA, Goodman KA, et al. Nonoperative management of rectal cancer with complete clinical response after neoadjuvant therapy. Ann Surg 2012;256(6):965–72.

55. De Caluwe L, Van Nieuwenhove Y, Ceelen WP. Preoperative chemoradiation versus radiation alone for stage II and III resectable rectal cancer. Cochrane Database Syst Rev 2013;(2):CD006041.

56. Braendengen M, Tveit KM, Bruheim K, et al. Late patient-reported toxicity after preoperative radiotherapy or chemoradiotherapy in nonresectable rectal cancer: results from a randomized Phase III study. Int J Radiat Oncol Biol Phys 2011;81(4):1017–24.

57. Ishihara S, Hayama T, Yamada H, et al. Benefit of tegafur-uracil and leucovorin in chemoradiotherapy for rectal cancer. Hepatogastroenterology 2011; 58(107–108):756–62.

58. Siegel R, Burock S, Wernecke KD, et al. Preoperative short-course radiotherapy versus combined radiochemotherapy in locally advanced rectal cancer: a multicentre prospectively randomised study of the Berlin Cancer Society. BMC Cancer 2009;9:50.

59. Thong MS, Mols F, Lemmens VE, et al. Impact of chemotherapy on health status and symptom burden of colon cancer survivors: a population-based study. Eur J Cancer 2011;47(12):1798–807.

60. Bohm G, Kirschner-Hermanns R, Decius A, et al. Anorectal, bladder, and sexual function in females following colorectal surgery for carcinoma. Int J Colorectal Dis 2008;23(9):893–900.

61. Ellis R, Smith A, Wilson S, et al. The prevalence of erectile dysfunction in post-treatment colorectal cancer patients and their interests in seeking treatment: a cross-sectional survey in the west-midlands. J Sex Med 2010;7(4 Pt 1): 1488–96.

62. Hendren SK, O'Connor BI, Liu M, et al. Prevalence of male and female sexual dysfunction is high following surgery for rectal cancer. Ann Surg 2005;242(2): 212–23.

63. Breukink SO, van Driel MF, Pierie JP, et al. Male sexual function and lower urinary tract symptoms after laparoscopic total mesorectal excision. Int J Colorectal Dis 2008;23(12):1199–205.

64. Quah HM, Jayne DG, Eu KW, et al. Bladder and sexual dysfunction following laparoscopically assisted and conventional open mesorectal resection for cancer. Br J Surg 2002;89(12):1551–6.

65. Stamopoulos P, Theodoropoulos GE, Papailiou J, et al. Prospective evaluation of sexual function after open and laparoscopic surgery for rectal cancer. Surg Endosc 2009;23(12):2665–74.

66. Ho VP, Lee Y, Stein SL, et al. Sexual function after treatment for rectal cancer: a review. Dis Colon Rectum 2011;54(1):113–25.

67. Maas CP, Moriya Y, Steup WH, et al. A prospective study on radical and nerve-preserving surgery for rectal cancer in the Netherlands. Eur J Surg Oncol 2000; 26(8):751–7.

68. Tekkis PP, Cornish JA, Remzi FH, et al. Measuring sexual and urinary outcomes in women after rectal cancer excision. Dis Colon Rectum 2009;52(1):46–54.

69. Schmidt CE, Bestmann B, Kuchler T, et al. Impact of age on quality of life in patients with rectal cancer. World J Surg 2005;29(2):190–7.

70. Lange MM, van de Velde CJ. Urinary and sexual dysfunction after rectal cancer treatment. Nat Rev Urol 2011;8(1):51–7.

71. Morino M, Parini U, Allaix ME, et al. Male sexual and urinary function after laparoscopic total mesorectal excision. Surg Endosc 2009;23(6):1233–40.

72. Hendren SK, Swallow CJ, Smith A, et al. Complications and sexual function after vaginectomy for anorectal tumors. Dis Colon Rectum 2007;50(6):810–6.

73. Jayne DG, Brown JM, Thorpe H, et al. Bladder and sexual function following resection for rectal cancer in a randomized clinical trial of laparoscopic versus open technique. Br J Surg 2005;92(9):1124–32.

74. Yang L, Yu YY, Zhou ZG, et al. Quality of life outcomes following laparoscopic total mesorectal excision for low rectal cancers: a clinical control study. Eur J Surg Oncol 2007;33(5):575–9.

75. Asoglu O, Matlim T, Karanlik H, et al. Impact of laparoscopic surgery on bladder and sexual function after total mesorectal excision for rectal cancer. Surg Endosc 2009;23(2):296–303.

76. Kim JY, Kim NK, Lee KY, et al. A comparative study of voiding and sexual function after total mesorectal excision with autonomic nerve preservation for rectal cancer: laparoscopic versus robotic surgery. Ann Surg Oncol 2012;19(8): 2485–93.

77. Havenga K, Maas CP, DeRuiter MC, et al. Avoiding long-term disturbance to bladder and sexual function in pelvic surgery, particularly with rectal cancer. Semin Surg Oncol 2000;18(3):235–43.

78. Maurer CA. Urinary and sexual function after total mesorectal excision. Recent Results Cancer Res 2005;165:196–204.

79. Nishizawa Y, Ito M, Saito N, et al. Male sexual dysfunction after rectal cancer surgery. Int J Colorectal Dis 2011;26(12):1541–8.

80. Kyo K, Sameshima S, Takahashi M, et al. Impact of autonomic nerve preservation and lateral node dissection on male urogenital function after total mesorectal excision for lower rectal cancer. World J Surg 2006;30(6):1014–9.

81. Akasu T, Sugihara K, Moriya Y. Male urinary and sexual functions after mesorectal excision alone or in combination with extended lateral pelvic lymph node dissection for rectal cancer. Ann Surg Oncol 2009;16(10):2779–86.

82. Engel J, Kerr J, Schlesinger-Raab A, et al. Quality of life in rectal cancer patients: a four-year prospective study. Ann Surg 2003;238(2):203–13.

83. Col C, Hasdemir O, Yalcin E, et al. Sexual dysfunction after curative radical resection of rectal cancer in men: the role of extended systematic lymph-node dissection. Med Sci Monit 2006;12(2):CR70–4.

84. Cornish JA, Tilney HS, Heriot AG, et al. A meta-analysis of quality of life for abdominoperineal excision of rectum versus anterior resection for rectal cancer. Ann Surg Oncol 2007;14(7):2056–68.

85. Guren MG, Eriksen MT, Wiig JN, et al. Quality of life and functional outcome following anterior or abdominoperineal resection for rectal cancer. Eur J Surg Oncol 2005;31(7):735–42.

86. Sideris L, Zenasni F, Vernerey D, et al. Quality of life of patients operated on for low rectal cancer: impact of the type of surgery and patients' characteristics. Dis Colon Rectum 2005;48(12):2180–91.

87. Allal AS, Gervaz P, Gertsch P, et al. Assessment of quality of life in patients with rectal cancer treated by preoperative radiotherapy: a longitudinal prospective study. Int J Radiat Oncol Biol Phys 2005;61(4):1129–35.

88. Vironen JH, Kairaluoma M, Aalto AM, et al. Impact of functional results on quality of life after rectal cancer surgery. Dis Colon Rectum 2006;49(5):568–78.

89. Marijnen CA, van de Velde CJ, Putter H, et al. Impact of short-term preoperative radiotherapy on health-related quality of life and sexual functioning in primary rectal cancer: report of a multicenter randomized trial. J Clin Oncol 2005; 23(9):1847–58.

90. Lange MM, Maas CP, Marijnen CA, et al. Urinary dysfunction after rectal cancer treatment is mainly caused by surgery. Br J Surg 2008;95(8):1020–8.

91. Mannaerts GH, Schijven MP, Hendrikx A, et al. Urologic and sexual morbidity following multimodality treatment for locally advanced primary and locally recurrent rectal cancer. Eur J Surg Oncol 2001;27(3):265–72.

92. Daniels IR, Woodward S, Taylor FG, et al. Female urogenital dysfunction following total mesorectal excision for rectal cancer. World J Surg Oncol 2006; 4:6.

93. Kinugasa Y, Murakami G, Uchimoto K, et al. Operating behind Denonvilliers' fascia for reliable preservation of urogenital autonomic nerves in total mesorectal excision: a histologic study using cadaveric specimens, including a surgical experiment using fresh cadaveric models. Dis Colon Rectum 2006;49(7):1024–32.

94. Moriya Y. Function preservation in rectal cancer surgery. Int J Clin Oncol 2006; 11(5):339–43.

95. Pollack J, Holm T, Cedermark B, et al. Late adverse effects of short-course preoperative radiotherapy in rectal cancer. Br J Surg 2006;93(12):1519–25.

96. Baxter NN, Rothenberger DA, Lowry AC. Measuring fecal incontinence. Dis Colon Rectum 2003;46(12):1591–605.

97. Neuman HB, Schrag D, Cabral C, et al. Can differences in bowel function after surgery for rectal cancer be identified by the European Organization for Research and Treatment of Cancer quality of life instrument? Ann Surg Oncol 2007;14(5):1727–34.

98. Emmertsen KJ, Laurberg S. Low anterior resection syndrome score: development and validation of a symptom-based scoring system for bowel dysfunction after low anterior resection for rectal cancer. Ann Surg 2012;255(5):922–8.

99. Whistance RN, Conroy T, Chie W, et al. Clinical and psychometric validation of the EORTC QLQ-CR29 questionnaire module to assess health-related quality of life in patients with colorectal cancer. Eur J Cancer 2009;45(17):3017–26.

100. Kneist W, et al. Is intraoperative neuromonitoring associated with better functional outcome in patients undergoing open TME?: Results of a case-control study. Eur J Surg Oncol 2013;39(9):994–9.

101. Kneist W, Junginger T. Male urogenital function after confirmed nerve-sparing total mesorectal excision with dissection in front of Denonvilliers' fascia. World J Surg 2007;31(6):1321–8.

102. Hanna NN, Guillem J, Dosoretz A, et al. Intraoperative parasympathetic nerve stimulation with tumescence monitoring during total mesorectal excision for rectal cancer. J Am Coll Surg 2002;195(4):506–12.

103. Laforest A, Bretagnol F, Mouazan AS, et al. Functional disorders after rectal cancer resection: does a rehabilitation programme improve anal continence and quality of life? Colorectal Dis 2012;14(10):1231–7.

104. Devroede G, Giese C, Wexner SD, et al. Quality of life is markedly improved in patients with fecal incontinence after sacral nerve stimulation. Female Pelvic Med Reconstr Surg 2012;18(2):103–12.

105. Faucheron JL, Chodez M, Boillot B. Neuromodulation for fecal and urinary incontinence: functional results in 57 consecutive patients from a single institution. Dis Colon Rectum 2012;55(12):1278–83.

106. Schwandner O. Sacral neuromodulation for fecal incontinence and "low anterior resection syndrome" following neoadjuvant therapy for rectal cancer. Int J Colorectal Dis 2013;28(5):665–9.

107. Breukink SO, van der Zaag-Loonen HJ, Bouma EM, et al. Prospective evaluation of quality of life and sexual functioning after laparoscopic total mesorectal excision. Dis Colon Rectum 2007;50(2):147–55.

108. Heriot AG, Tekkis PP, Fazio VW, et al. Adjuvant radiotherapy is associated with increased sexual dysfunction in male patients undergoing resection for rectal cancer: a predictive model. Ann Surg 2005;242(4):502–10 [discussion: 510–1].

109. Lindsey I, Mortensen NJ. Iatrogenic impotence and rectal dissection. Br J Surg 2002;89(12):1493–4.

110. Sterk P, Shekarriz B, Gunter S, et al. Voiding and sexual dysfunction after deep rectal resection and total mesorectal excision: prospective study on 52 patients. Int J Colorectal Dis 2005;20(5):423–7.

111. Donovan KA, Thompson LM, Hoffe SE. Sexual function in colorectal cancer survivors. Cancer Control 2010;17(1):44–51.

112. Pettit PD, Chen A. Implantable neuromodulation for urinary urge incontinence and fecal incontinence: a urogynecology perspective. Urol Clin North Am 2012;39(3):397–404.

113. Herbison GP, Arnold EP. Sacral neuromodulation with implanted devices for urinary storage and voiding dysfunction in adults. Cochrane Database Syst Rev 2009;(2):CD004202.

An Approach to the Newly Diagnosed Colorectal Cancer Patient with Synchronous Stage 4 Disease

Frederick Denstman, MD*

KEYWORDS

- Colorectal cancer • Stage 4 disease • Metastatic • Synchronous

KEY POINTS

- Evidence of stage 4 disease should give the surgeon reason to pause and evaluate carefully with an aim to develop an individualized treatment plan.
- Although algorithmic diagrams are popular as aids to treatment plans in medicine, stage 4 colorectal cancer is probably too complex for diagrams. There are too many variables.
- The surgeon should know that although most patients with colorectal cancer with stage 4 disease will ultimately die from their cancer, there is a significant number of patients who can be palliated in a meaningful way, and a very small number who may actually be cured.
- The surgeon along with his colleagues needs to carefully select patients who can be palliated and those who may be cured from the larger group to ensure optimal care.
- Some patients should never see the inside of an operating room except perhaps for the implantation of an intravenous chemotherapy port.

Eighty percent of patients with colorectal cancer (CRC) present with local or regional disease. For these patients, the general plan of treatment is clear: surgery with the intent of cure. However, about 20% of newly diagnosed patients continue to present with synchronously diagnosed stage 4 disease. For these patients, the treatment plan is less obvious. Despite their advanced stage of disease, a subset of stage 4 patients are potentially curable. This subset is of patients with so-called oligometastasis. The rest of these patients have truly disseminated disease and cannot be cured. Some patients with disseminated disease declare their condition immediately. Others patients with disseminated disease may at first masquerade as potentially curable metastatic disease, only to blossom into full-blown disseminated disease later in their course. The current staging system does not address these subsets.

Helen F. Graham Cancer Center, Christiana Care Health System, Newark, DE, USA
* Colon and Rectal Surgery Associates of Delaware, 4745 Stanton-Ogletown Road, Suite 216, Newark, DE 19713.
E-mail address: fdenstman@gmail.com

Surg Oncol Clin N Am 23 (2014) 151–160
http://dx.doi.org/10.1016/j.soc.2013.09.013
1055-3207/14/$ – see front matter © 2014 Elsevier Inc. All rights reserved.
surgonc.theclinics.com

The problem the surgeon faces in treating these stage 4 CRC patients is to try to identify the burden of metastatic disease and to provide an appropriate treatment plan. Patients with minimal metastatic disease that is potentially treatable for cure or long-term survival should be offered aggressive treatment. The approach is usually resection of both the primary and the metastatic tumor. Conversely, patients with disseminated disease should not undergo surgery if it offers no chance of cure or meaningful palliation.

When faced with synchronous stage 4 disease, the surgeon must develop a treatment plan that addresses whether to proceed directly to surgery, and if so, what operation or operations should be performed and in what order; whether to recommend chemotherapy and/or radiation therapy first and then re-evaluate; or whether to avoid surgery altogether in favor of long-term chemotherapy or a hospice approach.

Because there are so many different types and degrees of metastatic disease, and because the primary bowel tumors present in various ways, the decision-making process for these patients can be complex. These patients are not easily categorized and their treatment plans defy development of precise algorithms. Treatment of these patients requires more judgment than perhaps any other form of cancer. Multidisciplinary input is helpful. This input includes experts in medical and radiation oncology as well as diagnostic and interventional radiology. Input from surgeons with expertise in surgery of the large bowel, liver, lung, and occasionally other organs may be required.

One approach to planning treatment of a new patient with colon and rectal cancer is to answer a series of questions:

- Does the patient have synchronous metastatic disease?
- Is immediate surgery required for palliation of the primary tumor?
- What is the type and extent of metastatic disease?
- Is the metastatic disease amenable to potentially curative surgery?
- Should the metastatic disease be treated before the primary disease?
- If the patient is not curable, is there an opportunity for meaningful prolongation of life by either surgical or nonsurgical measures?

DOES THE PATIENT HAVE SYNCHRONOUS STAGE 4 CANCER?

The first suspicion of metastatic disease may arise during the history and physical examination. However, most metastatic disease is first identified by staging investigations. Computed tomographic (CT) scan of the chest, abdomen, and pelvis has several advantages. Good equipment is widely available and not operator dependent. Radiologists skilled in interpreting the study are also widely available. The study provides information for planning a resection and will generally confirm the location of the tumor.

CT scan is an excellent study for examining the liver, the most common site of distant metastasis. Ideally the study should include both arterial and portal phases of intravenous contrast. A noncontrast CT scan has poor sensitivity for detecting small liver lesions. Occasionally contrast will be omitted because of contrast allergy or simply deferred based on patient preference or issues with intravenous access. In these cases the surgeon should decide how critical it is to delay surgery in favor of better imaging. Options are to repeat the CT study of the liver with contrast, or to consider a complementary study such as magnetic resonance imaging or ultrasound.

Magnetic resonance imaging with contrast is comparable to or better than CT scan with some advantages, such as better specificity for benign liver lesions and more precise demarcation of intrahepatic vascular anatomy. It is also superior for evaluating response to preresection chemotherapy.[1] Because this test is longer, more uncomfortable, and more expensive, it is usually not ordered routinely. Ultrasound in highly skilled hands is also of some value, but this is highly operator dependent and, because the cross-sectional imaging studies have gained greater sophistication, ultrasound has become a less important tool. Its main use now is as an intraoperative study, performed by the surgeon during hepatic resection.

In the past a standard posteroanterior and lateral chest radiograph was considered to be an adequate preliminary tool for identification of lung metastases. More recently, inclusion of chest CT has gained favor. Many of the small, nonspecific parenchymal lesions that show up on chest CT turn out to be of no clinical significance, creating distractions for the medical team and anxiety for the patient. These small nonspecific CT scan lesions in a patient with a normal chest radiograph are often benign and should not play a major role in operative planning.

Positron emission tomography should not be a routine initial staging tool for CRC patients. At this time, positron emission tomography should mainly be used to help define equivocal CT scan findings, and before aggressive surgery for metastatic disease, such as major hepatic or pulmonary resection.

IS IMMEDIATE SURGERY REQUIRED FOR PALLIATION OF THE PRIMARY TUMOR?

Although the presence of the synchronous metastasis is ominous, 3 tumor characteristics trump the immediate concerns about the distant tumor spread: obstruction, bleeding, and pain due to invasion of local structures.

In this clinical context, obstruction is the presence of cramps, abdominal distension, nausea, vomiting, constipation, or the passage of frequent loose stools. One should probably not include asymptomatic patients who are described as being "obstructed" by the endoscopist because of an inability to pass a colonoscope through the lesion. Some of these "endoscopic obstructions" include patients who may go for many months before developing symptoms, which is especially true of lesions proximal to the splenic flexure where the stool is liquid.

For patients with bona fide high-grade obstruction, the best course of action is usually operative. Although chemotherapy or radiation therapy may reduce the size of the primary tumor, the therapeutic benefits are at best slow to occur. In the truly obstructed patient with stage 4 CRC, there are 4 options: resection with primary anastomosis; resection with end stoma; proximal diversion or bypass without resection; or placement of an endoluminal stent or other endoluminal therapy. Ideally, the lesion can be resected, but the exact strategy will be determined by the patient's general state of health.

On first impression, endoscopic placement of an endoluminal stent seems quite attractive. The advantages of this procedure are complete avoidance of a surgical incision or general anesthesia. However stenting has several limitations. The technique can be difficult and is not widely practiced. There is a risk of perforation, either during insertion or as a delayed complication. The luminal diameter of the stent is relatively small compared with the normal colon. When inserted into the left side of the colon, where stool is normally solid, the patient must be attentive to maintaining a liquid stool to prevent obstruction of the stent by solid stool. This maintenance has been compared with being on a perpetual bowel preparation for the patient. Finally, the stent cannot be easily used for low rectal cancers because of the tendency for the distal tip of the stent to create severe tenesmus or occasionally extrude through the anal canal. Stent migration can occur. Nevertheless stenting is appropriate in a small subset of patients. Other techniques such as laser fulguration are even less widely practiced.

Less commonly a large endophytic colon cancer may invade an adjacent loop of small bowel, causing a small bowel obstruction. This form of obstruction must be carefully differentiated from a colon obstruction. Obviously a proximal colostomy or endoluminal stent would do nothing to alleviate this obstruction, putting the patient through an unnecessary and ineffective surgical or endoluminal procedure. In these cases a direct surgical approach to the tumor is required.

In patients with heavily bleeding cancers, surgical resection may be the only way to prevent the need for frequent transfusions, even in incurable stage 4 disease. This bleeding can be particularly bothersome if the patient has a requirement for long-term anticoagulation with warfarin, heparin, clopidogrel, or any of the growing number of new potent anticoagulants. In this setting, simple diversion or bypass will likely not stop the bleeding.

When considering anemia as an indication for immediate surgery, the surgeon must consider the type of bleeding. Anemia is a common presenting finding in CRC patients, particularly with right colon cancers. Most of these patients present with an iron deficiency anemia that has developed insidiously. This anemia must be distinguished from the previously described pattern of acute lower gastrointestinal bleeding. Although initial correction of severe anemia may require transfusion, the need for ongoing transfusions may be obviated with daily oral iron replacement and urgent resection is generally not needed.

Pain caused by aggressive T4 invasion of adjacent structures by the tumor may be another indication for early resection in synchronous stage 4 CRC, including patients in whom a large tumor is invading the parietes, causing somatic pain. Before attempting resection, the surgeon should be confident that an R0 excision can be achieved. Leaving tumor behind will likely do nothing to alleviate the somatic pain. The classic example of an unresectable tumor would be sacral or deep pelvic side wall invasion by a rectal cancer. In these patients, pain usually indicates that the tumor is unresectable by conventional techniques.

If none of these urgent indications for surgery are present in the stage 4 patient, then the surgeon should consider whether the patient would be better served initially by a nonoperative approach. These decisions are probably best approached on a multidisciplinary level, ideally in the setting of a multidisciplinary cancer conference.

WHAT IS THE TYPE AND EXTENT OF METASTATIC DISEASE?

If preoperative staging fails to identify metastatic disease, the surgeon should generally proceed directly to surgery. An exception to this is locally advanced distal rectal cancer in which neoadjuvant chemoradiotherapy or short-course preoperative radiotherapy may be used.

Certain forms of metastatic disease continue to elude imaging studies, such as early carcinomatosis and subcentimeter metastatic nodules, so surgeons must perform a careful exploration of the peritoneal cavity at the beginning of every case. These unexpected findings call for an intraoperative judgment to change the surgical plan.

Extensive local or regional metastasis may be suspected because of history and physical examination and is usually confirmed by imaging studies. This form of metastasis is frequently a more challenging surgical problem than distant metastasis. For cancers of the colon or upper rectum, the surgeon should consider whether the regional disease will prevent a complete resection of the tumor. Where an en bloc resection seems possible, surgery should proceed. In the abdomen this could include resection of adjacent organs, such as body wall, neighboring loops of bowel, kidney, liver, stomach, spleen, and pancreas. In the pelvis, this could include more problematic en bloc resections involving sacrum, bladder, prostate, uterus, and ureters. Here the postponement of surgery in favor neoadjuvant therapy may offer some advantage.

Except to stem hemorrhage or relieve obstruction, a surgeon should avoid beginning a surgical resection, which is likely to end with residual gross tumor. Where an R0 resection appears to be uncertain, referral to a more experienced or specialized surgeon is appropriate.

Distant metastatic disease requires a different approach. The term "synchronous metastatic disease" is actually a misnomer, because virtually all metastatic events, regardless of when they present, have implanted before the detection of the primary tumor. However, when metastatic disease is detectable from the very beginning, it is more ominous because it immediately announces a more aggressive natural history of the patient's cancer. Even in cases where the synchronous disease seems "limited," the fact there is any visible metastatic disease portends the potential presence of numerous microscopic foci of disease, which will soon blossom into macroscopic disease.

APPROACH TO STAGE 4 CRC TO THE LIVER

Unfortunately most patients with synchronous liver metastases have incurable disease and resection of the primary tumor may not be the best step. Patients with obstruction, hemorrhage, and certain types of pain will usually be improved by initial resection of the primary, but in patients with extensive metastatic disease, the surgeon should look for ways to avoid surgery in favor of palliative chemotherapy or other palliative care.

One of the first steps in approaching patients with synchronous liver disease is to separate the incurable from the potentially curable. Although the number of patients who qualify for liver resection is still relatively small, the indications have increased significantly over the last 10 years or so. This increase is due to several advances. The first is the general improvement in liver resection techniques that have greatly reduced the risk of major hepatic resection and has tipped the risk:benefit ratio in favor of resection. These advances include the use of "low CVP" anesthesia, better training of hepatic surgeons, better preoperative and intraoperative imaging modalities, and techniques such as portal vein embolization[2] and 2-stage hepatic resections.[3] Although the morbidity of major resections is still fairly high (20%–50%), the mortality in large centers is less than 5%. Furthermore, the use of chemotherapy as a type of "adjuvant" therapy to hepatic resection, although still controversial, gives additional hope to these patients. It seems to offer at least some improvement in progression-free survival.

In the past, the presence of more than 4 intrahepatic lesions and the presence of bilobar disease were considered contraindications to hepatic resection; this is no longer true. The only universally agreed on contraindications now are (1) inability to perform an R0 resection and (2) the inability to preserve a remnant liver volume adequate to support life. However, this is not an automatic pass for every patient where the above 2 conditions are met. For example, synchronous liver disease by itself is a poor prognostic indicator. There are also a number or other poor prognostic indicators, any of which when taken alone may not contraindicate surgery, but when present in combination with enough other poor predictors may so mitigate the likelihood of success that a resection should not be offered.

There is still controversy over other absolute contraindications. Although many resectionists still view the presence of most types of extrahepatic metastatic disease, especially peritoneal carcinomatosis and aortocaval lymphadenopathy as strong contraindications, trials have indicated that some forms of extrahepatic disease, if effectively extirpated, may still allow for liver resection.

Therefore, when evaluating synchronous stage 4 CRC, it behooves the surgeon caring for the colon primarily not to exclude the patient from an aggressive effort simply because of the presence of liver lesions. Rather, the bowel surgeon should realize that hepatic resection is the standard of care for isolated or minimal liver metastases. Even very large, imposing lesions in the liver may be manageable in the hands of an experienced hepatic surgeon. When encountering synchronous stage 4 liver disease, the bowel surgeon should not be deterred from looking for a curative plan if the liver disease is potentially curable. In the best scenario, an isolated hepatic metastasis will rarely deprive the chance for cure. In the worst scenario, diffuse multisegmental disease will almost always rule out a cure. Many patients occupy the middle ground, and this is where consultation with an experienced hepatic surgeon will be needed to construct an overall treatment plan (**Box 1**).

Practically speaking, most patients with synchronous metastatic disease will never qualify for liver directed surgery with curative intent. Even in the small subset of patients who are offered hepatic resection, the concept of "potential cure" must be placed in careful context. Although numerous series show survival rates of 25% to 35%, after liver resection, the fine print indicates that these figures include survivors with detectable active disease, with only a very small cohort of survivors with no evidence of disease. To be sure, for those patients who qualify for resection of metastases, resection is the only hope for cure and this should be the goal of these resections. Far too often, though, metastases recur in the remnant liver, or in other sites, especially in the lungs. There is even a well-proven role for repeat liver resection or lung resection in a small subset of these recurrences, with rare but real long-term survivals.

Box 1
Unfavorable prognostic indicators for liver resection in metastatic CRC

Absolute contraindications

   Inability to obtain an R0 margin in the liver

   Unresectable extrahepatic disease

   Inability to preserve an adequate liver remnant

Poor prognostic indicators

   Synchronous metastasis

   Disease interval less than 1 y

   Metastatic tumor greater than 5 cm

   Carcinoembryonic antigen greater than 200

   Node-positive primary tumor status (N1)

   Hepatic portal node positive

   Resectable extrahepatic disease

   Progression of colorectal metastases on aggressive chemotherapy

   Poor cardiovascular or renal status

   Poor remnant liver status (steatohepatitis, "chemoliver," cirrhosis)

   Microsatellite instability

Data from Jarnagin WR, editor. Blumgart's surgery of the liver, biliary tract and pancreas. Philadelphia: Elsevier; 2012. p. 1290–304.

When hepatic resection becomes part of the treatment plan, a decision must be made as to its timing and the order of therapeutic steps. The timing and order may be one of the most subjective and controversial parts of the treatment plan. One school of thought suggests that patients should undergo aggressive chemotherapy as a first step, before surgery on the liver or the primary tumor, as a way of allowing more time for additional sites of metastasis to be declared. Progression of metastatic disease during chemotherapy is a poor prognostic feature and, although most hepatic surgeons will still proceed if there is only minor progression, the appearance of multiple new nodules should generally be viewed as a contraindication. In these unfortunate cases, allowing this period of expectant management could potentially spare the patient unnecessary surgery. Another method of expectant liver management is to proceed directly to colon resection, putting the liver resection on hold. Then the liver can be monitored for the appearance of new disease, while the patient is given a month or 2 to recuperate from the bowel surgery. If the hepatic disease remains stable, it can be attacked.

Further controversy exists over when chemotherapy should be offered to patients undergoing liver resection as a sort of adjuvant or neoadjuvant therapy. This controversy is the subject of ongoing trials. Many hepatic surgeons advocate a short or medium course of FOLFOX (5-FU + leucovorin + oxaliplatin) of FOLFIRI (5-FU + leucovorin + irinotecan) before surgery, with completion of the full course after recovery from the liver surgery. Because there is some evidence that preoperative treatment increases operative morbidity, other surgeons prefer to deliver the entire chemotherapeutic course postoperatively.

This form of neoadjuvant therapy should be differentiated from the concept of "conversion chemotherapy." Conversion chemotherapy is reserved for patients with moderate disease who are thought to be unresectable based on the number or location of lesions, but also thought to be "borderline" between resectability and nonresectability in the sense that a slight decrease in the size of the lesions might make resection possible. Although the likelihood of success here is small, Bismuth and colleagues[4] were able to convert 16% of a selected group of initially unresectable patients to resectability, with respectable long-term results, thereby "converting" these livers.

A further decision about timing relates to how the liver surgery should be carried out with respect to resection of the primary. On the one hand, it would seem ideal to handle resection of both the primary tumor and the liver disease during the same operation, as may be practical, depending of the type of liver resection and colon resection required. Surgical teams are more likely to offer these combined resections when the liver resection is less extensive and the bowel surgery is less extensive. For example, combining a segmental colon resection with a resection of the left lateral liver segment seems reasonable in many patients. Combining a right hepatectomy with a more complex rectal cancer resection is rarely offered because of concerns regarding higher infection and transfusion rates, longer operative times, and higher levels of physiologic stress.

A relatively new modification in the timing of surgery with synchronous metastasis involves reversing the order of surgery, sometimes referred to as "flipping," or "liver-first" surgery. Usually resection of the primary either precedes or is performed simultaneously with the liver resection. However, cases occur whereby it seems prudent to perform the liver resection first, delaying the resection of the primary. The most common scenario is in the case where a patient presents with a locally advanced T3 or T4 low rectal cancer and a large hepatic metastasis near a critical vascular structure. The colon and rectal surgeon wants to precede his surgery by neoadjuvant chemoradiation therapy because he is concerned about margins or local recurrence in the pelvis. Unfortunately standard chemoradiation therapy for rectal cancer is minimally effective against liver lesions in most cases, and the hepatic surgeon is worried that during the long period of neoadjuvant therapy for the rectum, the hepatic lesion will grow to the point of unresectability. Furthermore, the hepatic surgeon argues that the patient is more likely to die from advancing metastatic disease than the local disease, especially when the rectal cancer surgeon feels he can ultimately perform an R0 resection of the primary. The medical oncologist suggests that he can treat both sites with FOLFOX or FOLFIRI, but the hepatic surgeon argues that if the lesion is resistant to even this more aggressive form of chemotherapy, he may lose his one opportunity to cure the liver disease. Analogous situations can arise with synchronous colon cancer as well. One solution to this problem is to "flip" the order of more traditional treatment by performing the liver surgery first. This flipping allows a more relaxed approach to treatment of the large bowel primary. This treatment has been offered to a small group of synchronous stage 4 patients with good initial results.[5]

APPROACH TO STAGE 4 CRC TO THE LUNG

The approach to patients with pulmonary metastasis is somewhat analogous to the approach to hepatic metastases. About 10% of CRC patients present with lung metastases, and only 10% of these patients have isolated lung metastases. Most of the remaining 90% also have hepatic involvement.

In the rare patient with minimal pulmonary involvement and no extrapulmonary metastatic disease, pulmonary resection is favored. The refinement of video-assisted thoracic surgery has made this more appealing. The number of patients eligible for pulmonary resection is even smaller than those for hepatic resection. As a result, the outcome for these patients is less well studied and it is difficult to derive statistically valid guidelines. More recent studies show a 30% to 40% 5-year survival in resected patients with limited pulmonary metastatic disease; however, this is not necessarily disease-free survival. Prognostic factors include the presence of disease in mediastinal lymph nodes, advanced age, male gender, larger number of pulmonary nodules, and short disease-free survival. Preoperative imaging studies are not sensitive for identifying mediastinal spread.[6,7]

Although patients with a combination of liver and lung metastases tend to have short survivals after resection, a small subset of these patients may still be eligible for resection. The past practice of simultaneous liver and lung resection has lost favor. One approach has been to address the liver first. If the liver can be completely cleared, the lungs can be addressed at a later time, assuming that the metastatic disease has not advanced prohibitively.

APPROACH TO STAGE 4 CRC TO THE PERITONEUM

Carcinomatosis is a vexing pattern of stage 4 CRC. Although very common in stage 4 disease, it is difficult to detect with preoperative staging studies except in its more pronounced stages.

Traditionally, the approach to carcinomatosis has been systemic chemotherapy. Modern systemic chemotherapy offers a mean survival of 22 months. Recent trials have looked at "debulking surgery" combined with hyperthermic intraperitoneal chemotherapy. Although the results of these trials have been greeted with enthusiasm in some centers, this therapy is still controversial. The morbidity and mortality of this treatment are considerable. The recovery time from surgery tends to be long. Patients with node-positive disease tend not to benefit. The subset of patients that show the greatest benefit are those with a complete gross clearance of tumor, a difficult if not impossible achievement in many patients. Nevertheless, this may be a worthwhile form of palliation in a small subset of CRC patients. Because of the planning required for this treatment, it typically occurs as a type of second-look procedure after an initial surgery for resection of the primary.[8]

Isolated ovarian metastases are rare and frequently portend disseminated disease. Ovarian involvement can occur as a form of limited carcinomatosis or via lymphatic spread. Abnormal ovaries should be removed with the primary tumor when possible. The presence of suspicious ovaries would rarely be reason enough to abort resection of the primary tumor.[9]

SUMMARY

Evidence of stage 4 disease should give the surgeon reason to pause and consider the patient's options carefully. These patients should be evaluated carefully with an aim to develop an individualized treatment plan. This individualized treatment plan requires input from other disciplines, optimally through a multidisciplinary cancer conference, and there should be good communication between the patient, the surgeon, and his or her colleagues.

Although algorithmic diagrams are popular as aids to treatment plans in medicine, stage 4 CRC is probably too complex for diagrams. There are too many variables. Stage 4 disease is an uphill climb. The surgeon should know that although most CRC patients with stage 4 disease will ultimately die from their cancer, there is a significant number of patients who can be palliated in a meaningful way, and a very small number who may actually be cured. The surgeon along with his colleagues needs to select these latter 2 groups of patients from the larger group to ensure optimal care. Conversely, some of these patients should never see the inside of an operating room except perhaps for the implantation of an intravenous chemotherapy port.

REFERENCES

1. Adams R, Aloai TA, Loyer E, et al. Selection for hepatic resection of colorectal liver metastases: expert consensus statement. HPB (Oxford) 2013;15:91–103.
2. Azoulay D, Castaing D, Smail A, et al. Resection of non-resectable liver metastases from colorectal cancer after percutaneous portal vein embolization. Ann Surg 2000;231:480–6.
3. Tsai S, Marques HP, Choti MA, et al. Two stage strategy for patients with extensive bilateral colorectal liver metastases. HPB (Oxford) 2010;12:262–9.
4. Bismuth H, Adam R, Levi F, et al. Resection of non-resectable liver metastases from colorectal cancer liver metastases after neoadjuvant chemotherapy. Ann Surg 1996;224:509–22.
5. deJong MC, VanDam RM, Dejung CH. The liver-first approach for synchronous colorectal liver metastases: a 5-year single center experience. HPB (Oxford) 2011;13:745–52.
6. Hamaji M, Cassivi SD, Shenk R, et al. Is lymph node dissection required in pulmonary metastasectomy for colorectal adenocarcinoma? Ann Thorac Surg 2012;94:1796–801.
7. Blackmon SH, Stephens EH, Correa AM, et al. Predictors of recurrent pulmonary metastases and survival after pulmonary metastasectomy for colorectal cancer. Ann Thorac Surg 2012;94:1802–9.

8. Verwaal VJ, Bruin S, Boot H, et al. Eight year follow-up of randomized trial cytor-eduction and hyperthermic intraperitoneal chemotherapy versus systemic chemotherapy in patients with peritoneal carcinomatosis of colorectal cancer. Ann Surg Oncol 2008;15:2426–32.

9. Beck DE, Roberts PL, Saclarides TJ, et al, editors. The ASCRS Textbook of colon and rectal surgery. New York: Springer; 2011. p. 796–7.

Index

Note: Page numbers of article titles are in **boldface** type.

A

Abdominoperineal excision, of rectal cancer, **93–111**
    current controversies in, 106–109
        extent of perineal dissection and removal of pelvic floor, 106–107
        positioning of patient for, 107–108
        reconstruction of pelvic floor, 108–109
    extralevator, 99–103
    intersphincteric, 99
    ischioanal, 103–106
    new concept of, 97–99
    problems with convention synchronous combined, 95–97
Adenomas, detection rate with colonoscopy, 3–4
    avoiding missed, 6–7
    reasons for missed, 4
Adjuvant chemotherapy, for colorectal cancer, **49–58**
    challenges and barriers to, 52–53
    importance of timing, 51–52
Age, and functional consequences of colorectal cancer management, 128–129, 133–134, 137
Anatomy, rectal, relevant to imaging in rectal cancer, 60–64
Antibiotics, prophylactic, in colon and rectal cancer surgery, 15–16

B

Bowel dysfunction, after treatment of colorectal cancer, 128–132
    colon cancer, 128
    patient factors, 128–129
    rectal cancer, 128
    treatment factors, 129–132
    tumor factors, 129

C

Cancer prevention, role of colonoscopy in, 2–3
Central vascular ligation, with complete mesocolic excision, 28–29
Chemoradiation, in rectal cancer, management of complete response after, **113–125**
    assessing response, 117–119
    defining complete response, 114
    future studies, 119–121
    interpreting the literature, 114–117
   neoadjuvant, of rectal cancer, controversies in, **79–92**
    choice of drugs and combination with radiation, 81–84

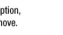

Printed and bound by CPI Group (UK) Ltd, Croydon, CR0 4YY

03/10/2024

01040409-0017